Built To Last

ABOUT THE AUTHOR

David Amerland has authored several influential books on SEO, including *Google Semantic Search*, which explores how Google's algorithm shifts to better understand user intent and deliver meaningful results. His work emphasizes the importance of context, relevance, and semantic connections in digital content strategies. By focusing on human-centric approaches, he has helped businesses adapt to the changing landscape of search and content marketing. Beyond SEO, Amerland's writings often delve into broader topics like decision-making, neuroscience, and the implications of artificial intelligence. Books like *The Sniper Mind* investigate the mental frameworks that lead to success in high-pressure environments, drawing parallels between military precision and business execution. A passionate martial artist he is a certified Tae Kwon Do Instructor, holds a 2nd degree Black Belt in ITF Tae Kwon Do, a Black Belt in WTF Tae Kwon Do, a Black Belt in Wado Ryu Karate and has had intermediate training in Kung Fu and Muay Thai. When he's not writing he's training.

Built To Last

How to Get Stronger, Healthier and Happier At
Every Stage of Life

David Amerland

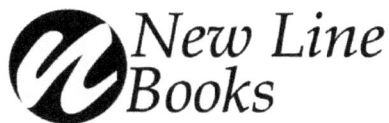

*New Line
Books*

FIRST EDITION

ISBN: 978-1-84481-183-0
eBook ISBN: 978-1-84481-184-7
Audiobook ISBN: 978-1-84481-185-4

A CIP catalogue reference for this book is available from the British Library.

This book contains advice and information relating to health care.
It should be used to supplement rather than replace the advice of your doctor
or another trained health professional. If you know or suspect you have a health
problem, it is recommended that you seek the advice of your physician or
any trained health professional you consult, before embarking on any treatment or
medical program. All efforts have been made to assure the accuracy of the
information contained in this book as of the date of publication. This publisher
and the author disclaim liability for any medical outcomes that may occur as a
result of applying the methods suggested in this book.

Every book has an origin story. This one owes its beginnings to George. Our conversations sparked the ideas that eventually made it happen. You know who you are. I cannot thank you enough!

ACKNOWLEDGEMENTS

There are a lot of people who have been part of this particular journey. Some input ideas. Others critiqued parts of this book. Some came with questions hoping that I can supply practical answers. The people in The Hive often became my navigation lights. Your struggles helped me narrow down some of the answers I give here, shedding the theoretical in favor of the practical. You are too many to mention by name, but thank you! DAREBEE provided the workouts and the illustrations helping expand the practical value of this book by orders of magnitude, transforming what would have been just another book on well-being into a standalone blueprint you can put to work from the very first chapter, to help you improve the health and strength of your body and brain. Bennie and Ollie kept an eye on me when I worked late and Neila made sure that however complex a task writing a book like this may be, I never felt alone.

TABLE OF CONTENTS

PREFACE

We all want the same basic things in life: to live long, stay healthy, and be happy. If we have those three, we can handle whatever challenges come our way.

But getting there can feel impossible—mainly because when we actually stop to think about it, we have no idea where to start. Breaking it all down into simple steps that we can act on isn't something we're taught to do. So instead, these big life goals seem so overwhelming that most of us just end up hoping for the best—wishing good health and happiness on ourselves and others during birthdays, holidays, and special occasions, as if the universe might grant them to us like a wish come true.

The truth is, we usually don't start thinking seriously about our health and well-being until something shakes us awake—a personal crisis, a health scare, or a reminder that the choices we make today shape our future long before life forces us to take control.

This book is here to help. It's not about magic solutions or one-size-fits-all formulas, because real health, fitness, and happiness are more complex than that. But at the same time, we all share the same biology, the same fundamental building blocks. And that's good news! It means there are universal principles we can use to improve our quality of life, feel better, live longer, and be happier.

The catch? It's up to you. No one is coming to do it for you, and no one will care if you do nothing. The responsibility is yours, no matter what stage of life you're in.

Each chapter in this book gives you a plan. Each plan includes actions. As you go through, you'll find the information you need to build your own approach—one that works for you.

And with the knowledge in these pages, along with the DAREBEE workouts included, you have everything you need to create a stronger, healthier, and happier life.

Make the most of it.

INTRODUCTION

Fitness is too important in life to be left to the lottery of socioeconomic status and zip code luck.

Whoever you are, wherever you are, you have a right to feel strong and be healthy all your life. Achieving this has to be your work, your construct, your project. For certain, you cannot do this without some help. None of us can.

This book addresses that.

Use it to feel stronger and be healthier. In the process you will become better than you ever thought you could be and feel happier than you imagined. Because of that it may also help you live longer, be more productive and achieve more of what you dream of.

Nothing would make me happier.

David

THE PARADOX OF FITNESS

Fitness is not what you have been led to believe it is. The only expert on your body is you and though you may, at times, seek outside specialized help the goals and the drive to get fit and stay healthy must come from you.

Think about being fit for a moment. What image comes to your mind? Depending on your age and sex I am going to bet that the images you project in your mental screen are people who are lean, sport a six pack and have strong and muscular arms and legs. While there may be a spectrum in just how specific and developed these attributes might be, these physical attributes are usually all present in the mental image we have of a fit person. And if I were to ask you a little more specifically about capabilities not just attributes then the mental model of a fit person you have created, in addition to looking lean and muscular is also capable of running fast, running long and jumping high for as long as possible.

Ask yourself now: Where did this image of a fit person come from? Certainly no one took you to one side one day, pulled up a chart and explained to you that fitness means this thing or that thing. Nor was it something you were taught specifically at home or at school in so many terms and so many visual images.

Our perception of what fitness is has come about by osmosis. We've absorbed it from our environment through a barrage of advertising images, fitness industry posters, what we see in magazines and what we see on our screens of professional athletes and the semi-naked images of film stars in major Hollywood films. All of these have contributed to our own mental image of what fitness is. What all these different industries have in common is the fact that whenever they promote an image of fitness that feeds into the popular conception of what fitness is, it is being promoted for professional reasons of their own that serve them and have nothing to do with what is actually good for us.

The paradox here, and it's an important one, lies in the fact that we all make the mistake of accepting an externally imposed and largely culturally guided idea of what fitness is. We then use that as a standard against which we measure our own. By doing so we, essentially, accept what the external world tells us about fitness and then we use that externally imposed definition to shape the unique internal world and physique of every individual to match it.

Obviously this can't work. If it did we wouldn't be having this discussion and you wouldn't be reading this book. You would already have the knowledge necessary and the understanding you need to help you be healthy and feel strong your entire life. And you would be practicing it.

A lot of what we will cover here appears intuitive. You already know it or sense it and if you don't citing numbers is not going to make much of a difference to how you really feel about it. We will look at some numbers however because when it comes to fitness, the numbers help create a clearer picture of the reality around us. It is the numbers that tell a grim story about the state of fitness of the people around us and, quite possibly, reflect part of our own directly experienced reality. And it is the numbers that help us better understand where we fit in the picture that is revealed.

A Gallup survey contacted in 2009, for example, found that nearly half (49%) of all Americans "report exercising for at least 30 minutes, less than three days per week." In other words nearly half the population of the United States exercises nowhere near enough to what it needs to so it can feel physically well and psychologically capable. We're not even examining specific fitness attributes like strength and endurance, we're only talking about basic exercise.

You'd think that a survey like that would be a strong wake-up call and something would have been done to change things, but no; the situation actually got worse. Nine years later, in 2018, the Center for Disease Control (CDC) and the Prevention National Center for Health Statistics (NCHS) drew on five years of data to show that only 23 per cent of Americans get enough exercise. That means that more than seven people out of ten do not exercise enough, if at all. In the intervening nine year gap between the first survey and the second half of the people who exercised, did so even less or had stopped.

Despite the fact that America leads the world in spending in every segment of the fitness market to the tune of $264.6 billion a year it ranks just 20th in participation in physical activities that are classed as exercise. The NCHS figures for 2020 showed that the number of Americans who got enough exercise had improved by barely one percentage point. Yet, in America alone the average consumer spends $111.80 per year on athletic gear and the fitness industry is poised to grow in terms of revenue, by approximately five per cent a year.

Globally the fitness industry is worth a staggering $828 billion. Yet what is spent on fitness gear is not reflected on improved effects on health or even in participation in exercise. In Europe, figures released by the Organization for Economic Cooperation and Development (OECD) for 2022 showed that more than one in three European adults does not do enough physical activity and only four in ten adults exercise regularly, with low rates in women, the elderly and lower socio-economic groups. This shows that despite all the socio-economic initiatives launched by European countries to help people exercise the number of people who don't do enough is six in ten, barely better than what we see in America.

Clearly, there is a disconnect here. We all understand the need for exercise and fitness. We are all willing to spend some money on it. But most of us are unwilling to actually exercise or, if we are, we appear unable to stick to it long enough for it to make a meaningful impact on our health and longevity.

The problem then, and this paradox makes it apparent, is not that we don't want to exercise or that we don't understand what exercise will give us. We just saw that we are bombarded from virtually all sides with ideal images of fit people. We are on the receiving end of constant reminders from government organizations and health authorities of the need to exercise and its benefits. We are constantly told by the advertising industry how important exercise is and why we need to spend money to get new shoes, new outfits, new equipment, new gym memberships. No, the real problem is that for reasons we will look at here, we can't make exercise an integral part of our lifestyle so that we can truly be healthier and live longer.

There are many reasons why this is happening. Each of them forms a layer of the paradox of fitness and we will unwrap them all, one by one. But let's start with a truism: our current setup of modern life makes good health difficult. It's a depressing thought and in this chapter we need to ask "Why?" Why is life as we currently experience it incompatible with good health? Surely the opposite should be true. Everything we do or, are told to do should be leading us to a healthier, longer life.

Even if we take the cynical approach that the world is a hard, cold, uncaring place that views each of us as a productive unit that's only there to work, earn money, consume goods and pay bills until we die, it stands to reason that it is to the world's benefit if we can do all these things it asks of us, with more vigor and for a longer time. And for that to happen however we need to be in good health and feel happy in our body.

Unfortunately this is not the reality most people experience as they age. The reason their experience is so different from the idealized version that we hold in our imagination should become evident as we peel back the layers of the fitness paradox to better understand what lies at its core.

No One Is In Charge

If you were an intrepid alien looking for some great intergalactic investment opportunities and came to planet Earth you too may want to invest in some of the organic, biomechanical units living there. You may reason that unlike on your planet where no one works because smart machines do everything, on planet Earth the bulk of the work, both manual and mental is performed by organics.

Organics have a shelf-life however. As they age they begin to perform below expectation and then, eventually, break down and die. As a smart intergalactic investor then you may think that if you managed to somehow purchase a number of these organics and set them to work for you, in order to get the most out of your investment you will need to ensure that each of them is guided by a nutritionist, a therapist and a personal trainer. That way not only will you prolong their lifespan and help them live longer so you can recoup your investment but you will also prolong their healthspan so they can work harder and help you turn a tidy profit.

To the best of my knowledge there are no aliens purchasing humans. The world also doesn't automatically provide us with nutritionists, personal trainers and therapists from the moment we are born so we can be healthier and live longer. The world, as we perceive it, appears not to care much about us because it is not an actual organized construct that has some kind of overseeing authority guiding it. The world emerges as a necessity that makes the many activities we engage in, as a species, possible.

As an emergent phenomenon, a wrapper of sorts, the world around us exists but it is not guided by anything beyond the blind dynamic forces that shape it. These forces are always reactive. Because they tend to shut the figurative stable door only after the horse has bolted, they help to highlight the magnitude of the problem but never really offer much of a solution until after the fact by which time everything is way harder to solve.

Let's take a look, however, at some figures to see just how that reactive nature takes form: In the World Health Organization (WHO) European Region report, being overweight and being obese affect almost 60% of adults and nearly one in three children (29% of boys and 27% of girls). The USA currently ranks first in obesity prevalence levels, Europe is in second place globally.

By the time these figures emerge get processed and are accepted it is already too late. On the ground they translate into a reality where there are a lot of people like you and I who have not had sufficient guidance in what to eat, how to eat, how to exercise and how to think about food and exercise. This means we are likely to end up in the depressing obesity statistics. If we are obese or even if we are just overweight we are significantly more likely to suffer from disease and die earlier. Even worse, before we die we are likely to experience a significant segment of time during which our quality of life and our ability to feel capable and be productive, requirements essential to experiencing personal happiness, will be severely limited.

Even at that stage, however, we may not be a completely lost cause destined to be consigned to the scrap heap. The return to good health and a long and happy life is certainly possible if we change the way we move our body, start to take care of our nutrition and do some work on our selves so that our emotional regulation, and the life choices we make, improve.

When no one is in charge it means that there is no benevolent alien coming to invest in us so that we can work for him and be as productive as possible for as long as possible and be well looked after in the process. Since no one is coming to save us this means there is no one looking out for us. We need to be the ones who take charge of ourselves and we need to be the ones who look after ourselves.

While this makes eminent logical sense it is also extremely difficult to navigate correctly. As we shall see, what we need to help us do so is a good plan.

The Adversary Within

Think, for a moment, about all the help we didn't get when we needed it the most.

No one came to teach us about nutrition, exercise and mental health when we needed it. Our brain however is not designed to accept an information vacuum, so we learned what we could from the sources available to us: our parents, friends, the media, movies and TV and the culture around us. We learned this by watching and emulating, by working things out for ourselves using the limited experience we had and by making certain assumptions that to us appeared correct at the time.

At best this approach created a haphazard image in our mind where we think that fitness, longevity, health and happiness depend upon achieving specific physical attributes that require hard work and sacrifice and are the prerogative of the few who can afford the time and the expense required to achieve them. Top athletes, movie stars and celebrities can afford them. They are the ones who have sufficient spare money to buy the expertise they don't themselves have and sufficient spare time to achieve the results they want. The rest of us, we feel, are locked into the daily grind of our lives that leave us few options.

It doesn't help that as we struggle with all this there is a strident voice within us that criticizes our every achievement, undermines our every effort and constantly makes us feel that every time we put effort into improving our self and fail we have failed because we simply are not good enough, not successful enough, not wealthy enough, not worthy enough.

Why does this happen? What form or forms does this internal adversary we all carry take?

Well, in a perfect world we would be our own cheerleaders. We would formulate plans in our head, we would break those plans down into specific goals and milestones and we would then set about to achieve them, while working with whatever unique set of limitations we each faced. The fact that we don't do that speaks volumes about what truly drives us, how our motivation is formed and how ancient neurobiological systems within us, trip us up and cause us to fail before.

Let's take something as simple as weight for instance to use as an example. In its 2023 publication on the prevalence of overweight and obesity Eurostat, the statistical office of the European Union, responsible for publishing high-quality Europe-wide statistics and indicators that enable comparisons between countries and regions stated that: "Obesity is a serious public health problem as it significantly increases the risk of chronic diseases such as cardiovascular disease, type-2 diabetes, hypertension, coronary heart diseases and certain cancers."

It highlighted the fact that "one in six Europeans is obese and over 50% of adults are overweight." If this planet had been specifically engineered by smart aliens interested in earning a healthy return on their investment they would already have put in place in advance a global dietary system aimed at optimizing our fuel intake and performance. Because these smart, alien overseers do not exist we are left with an imperfect system where the food industry looks to maximize its profits from what we eat.

To do that it relies on food being addictive and to make it so it pulls the tripwire in our brain labeled "easy energy". Easy energy for the ancient mechanism that runs us is sugar. And sugar in the ancient world from which we all have come, was hard to come by. As a result we are hardwired to look for it and when we do find it the brain's mesolimbic dopamine system gets activated.

Our brain then releases dopamine which makes us feel really, really good about ourselves. This is not just our reward for having found sugar but also the brain's way of making sure that we continue to look for sugar in the near future.

What worked to our benefit in that ancient world our body was born in and shaped by makes zero sense in a modern world whose landscape is dotted by fast food outlets and supermarkets. Yet it is in the modern world that this mechanism is activated now and when it does so it exhibits one additional response: stimulation tolerance.

Imagine how amazing it must have seemed to our hunter-gatherer ancestors to come across a beehive and harvest some wild honey. Not only would they feel good while consuming all that easy energy they came across but also the dopamine hit in their brains must have been like the strongest feel-good drugs we can take today. That's how intense the stimulation they felt must have been.

For us however access to jars of honey, cans of sweetened condensed milk, bars of chocolate and tabs of ice-cream is so easy that our brain, in order to protect itself from this frequent intense level of stimulation, rewires its excitation threshold, raising it as a result. So we end up needing more and more of what excites us to feel the same level of intensity and 'happiness' we felt when we first consumed it.

That is the textbook definition of addiction. And our food industry that adds sugar and salt (the other high excitation stimulant we are hardwired to seek) in our food then condemns us to either seek foods that are ever higher in sugar and salt content or consume more and more of the same foods we eat so we can eat greater quantities of sugar and salt so we can feel the same level of excitation we felt before.

Add to this the fact that the other naturally occurring "easy energy" food that is available to us is fat you can immediately see how if I or you were owners of a food factory we would naturally want to produce something that was high in sugar, fat and salt content because whatever that product was it would sell a lot and make us rich.

It is easy sometimes to blame the global food industry for this and demand that governments do something about it through regulations and labeling of the food we consume and sure, governments, having realized the health problem caused by obesity have started to produce legislation concerning foods. In the European Union food labels have to display all their ingredients. That though is not enough to save us from ourselves.

It is we who need to realize just how our own response to sugar, fat and salt contained in our food traps us and take the action necessary to mitigate its harmful impact.

So, one form our internal opponent, "the enemy within" we all carry, takes is our body's natural response to physical stimulants contained in food which, if we let it, undermines our efforts to be slimmer and healthier. But that is not the only form the enemy within takes. There is also that insidious, constant inner critic, the constant negative voice in our head that tells us we can't do something because we are not strong enough, not good enough, not capable enough and we should just give up.

That too has a good reason to be there.

Ancient Coding In A Modern Game Map

Anybody who has ever played a video game is familiar with the concept of a game map. That's the environment that game programmers employ that determines the physics of the game world, constrains the capabilities of the game players and makes the game what it is.

Whenever that world is updated the characters, both NPC and avatars that represent a human also need to be upgraded to take advantage of everything it offers. In the video games world any changes that are made to the game environment go hand-in-hand with changes to the code of the video game characters. In the real world however things change in a much slower and way less synchronized way.

The code that runs our body is a lot older than the code of our very modern environment. And when the ancient code that helped us survive in the past runs in the modern world we live in, it often creates glitches that hold us back.

This is where that negative voice in our head comes in. The negative self-talk a lot of us hear playing out in our head belittles our sense of self-worth, diminishes our achievements and undermines any efforts we make to improve our self. And although each of these acts is destructive to us, it is actually designed to help us. Or rather, it was designed to help us in a world that was a lot more hostile to us than the one we currently live in. That was the old game map of the past and back then there were parts of it we shouldn't access if we wanted to survive. In a video game any parts of the environment we cannot access (or shouldn't) is magically blocked to us. In the real world there are no such safe guards so any constraint in our movement and motivation comes from that negative voice within us which was originally designed to safeguard us from harm.

In scientific circles this negative voice in our head is known as negativity bias and there are a number of current scientific theories that explain its presence. Some of the more well-known ones cite risk-detection and loss-aversion as the primary causes of this negativity bias in us. The survival of our ancestors hinged on spotting the Saber-toothed tiger hunting them before it could eat them. In that scenario those who took more risks or paid less attention to the environment ended up as meals to predators and did not get the opportunity to find a mate and pass on their genes, which means that those who did were more likely to have this negative voice playing out inside their head.

Similarly, those of our ancestors who suffered the fewest losses in resources lived long enough to procreate and have descendants and their descendants valued not-losing what they had more than delighting in something they gained.

Evolutionary biologists sometimes cite a slightly more complex, more generalized theory they call "Concave fitness-state hypothesis" which encompasses both the risk-detection and loss-aversion hypotheses and proposes that they fit within the greater arc of homeostasis (i.e. the energetic balance of our internal state).

Basically homeostasis is the inner state of balance that allows us to go through life without experiencing any system crash that renders us physically, mentally or psychologically unable to respond to the survival demands made on us by our environment. To achieve that, the hypothesis goes, we are actually hardwired to avoid any potential threat, potential loss or even a large potential reward that would demand from us an increase in the effort required to do what we do. Obviously, as an example, none of us want to be eaten by a Saber-toothed tiger so avoiding any situation that would place us in close proximity to one is a no-brainer. But doing something that would end up losing us, perhaps, some equipment or a nice area where we could camp would also make our life difficult and end up costing us more energy expenditure by way of effort required to stay alive than it should. So we avoid that, too. And gaining perhaps a massive area to live in, much bigger than we truly need, which would also increase the effort required from us to keep it safe is something we are hardwired to avoid, presumably because those who didn't had a harder daily life and didn't make it long enough to pass on their genes to the next generation.

The key point of all this complex theorizing that is based in both mathematics and paleobiology is that when it comes to getting your self fit unless you're a professional who's career requires it, the odds are stacked against you.

The struggle you feel is real. When you fail to show up at the gym class you signed up for, when you fail to maintain your daily schedule which you promised yourself you would, when you fail to eat right and sleep more. When you reach for the wrong foods and when you let yourself slump in front of your television looking for a brief respite from the pressures of life, it's not because you're weak. It is because you're alone. It is not a question of character, it is a question of vested interest in what is happening around you and the lack of a support network that would help you. It is not because of money or class, though both of these play a role in how fit you get and how healthy you can stay as you age, it is a question of not being able to go against your own ancient biology and the responses that are hardwired in you because there is no one to help you when you're on the brink. There is no one to support you when you're physically or mentally tired.

Put in the simplest English possible, the ancient programming of our body and mind, the ancient code that runs inside us was never meant for this modern world we are in.

So, the question now begs itself: What can you do?

What choices remain open to you? What routes of action can you embark on that will ensure that you stay as fit and strong and young and healthy, as you age, as the richest, best supported and most attended people on the planet?

Anything? Is there something you can do?

Luckily for you the answer is "yes!".

Start With A Goal And Add A Plan

By now you must have realized that if you possessed a strong desire to remain fit and healthy all your life and a tangible reason to pursue it, you would need access to a reasonable amount of funding to hire personal trainers, nutritionists and dietitians who would help you achieve your goal.

I am making a reasonable guess that you haven't got any of these people helping you achieve your goal but that doesn't mean that there is no other way to get what you want.

I've always believed that fitness is fundamental to life. It is conducive to happiness and it is key to success and it should be available to everyone as a right, not a privilege.

You shouldn't need to sacrifice your health in order to get some wealth, though that is exactly what often happens in life. You shouldn't be resigned to being overweight, losing mobility and experiencing any of the life-debilitating and, occasionally, life-threatening conditions that are experienced by nearly one third of the global population, because they don't exercise.

Nor should you be resigned to feeling bad inside your own body because your inactivity and poor nutrition have created physical conditions that cause you discomfort and pain.

A WHO report that tracked levels of physical activity of adults across the world showed that in the twelve year period between 2010 and 2022 the number of adults who exercised dropped by 5% across the entire world. Approximately 1.8 billion people did not meet the recommended levels of physical activity in 2022, that's 31% of the world's population. If the trend remains unchecked it means that by 2030 over 35% of adults globally will not be doing sufficient exercise to remain healthy. As a result many of them will suffer from cardiovascular diseases such as heart attacks, strokes and type 2 diabetes. Their brain will deteriorate with age like any other organ in their body and they will be candidates for dementia plus they will be more likely to develop serious diseases such as breast and colon cancer. Their lifespan will be shortened and the quality of life of their later years will be significantly degraded robbing them of the basic right to simply enjoy being alive.

We have the data. We know the figures. We are totally aware of the effects. So why isn't something being done about it?

The fact is that while this problem is global the world is still a fragmented place where nations are regional and the policies they need to put in place have to be local. Somewhere between the grim global picture the figures show and the initiatives being put into effect in small communities at a local level in mostly developed countries, the sense of urgency is lost. Other imperatives jump the queue and command attention.

As I've said already no one is in charge. There are initiatives but no overarching plan. Authorities and those in power respond to the figures but never act pre-emptively.

This situation, in turn, leads to the epiphany that since no one is in charge of our health, both external and internal, it is up to you, up to us, each of us; to take charge of our own fitness journey in life and control the arc of our own personal physical and psychological development. To achieve this we need a goal, but as the French poet, journalist and aviator, Antoine de Saint-Exupéry famously said: "A goal without a plan is just a wish." So, what we need is a plan.

Like all good plans this one starts with you answering a few basic questions about yourself and being as honest as possible in the process. It will be helpful if you wrote your answers down somewhere, especially if you're reading this book as an ebook or listening to it as an audiobook. On the paperback you could potentially scribble on the margins or if there is some space, at the end of this chapter. Either way, by recording your answers and maybe also dating them, you will have a reminder of where you were in your fitness journey when you started and a handy reference point to help you better understand just how far you've come when the time comes for you to look at it, again.

For the plan to work we must start with the nearly invisible parts which are your mind and your heart. We must start, in other words, with what you think and how you feel.

For instance, it's not enough to articulate your goal by writing down "I want rock-hard abs" if you have no idea why you truly want them in the first instance and how you will feel about all the hard work required to get them and then maintain them.

To make this work, goals need to be articulated clearly and be realistic and feelings have to be considered with care. For example, if you have to lose 60 lbs, approximately 27 kg, going for "rock hard abs" as your stated goal is possible but improbable. The target is too far away and the effort required to get you there way too much to sustain for long, which makes it unrealistic.

On a perfect day when everything is going your way you may be able to pull off some really hard training but when you're having a bad day it's more than likely you will let things slide. That's a slippery slope that always ends with you quitting your fitness journey altogether and then having to deal with feelings of personal guilt and personal failure that are associated with the fact that you quit.

To avoid all this we're going to break down the plan you need into three very accessible stages, much like the intention to cook a meal. Before we start to prepare some type of food for ourselves we usually have a clear understanding of its intent: is what we're preparing intended to satisfy our hunger, in which case it is most likely savory or satisfy a craving, in which case it is most probably sweet. Is it going to be the main meal of the day and therefore needs to be relatively large and maybe complex or is it going to be a snack of sorts in which case it needs to be light and simple.

Everything from here on until will follows the law of threes, where three elements need to be pulled together to make something work.

The first stage of our plan is the formula we apply in order to break down its composition. Our fitness plan composition has three distinct elements in it and they are:

- Goal
- Ingredients
- Execution

Fitness Plan Goal

For 'Goal' you start with this in mind: whatever you aim for, it has to be reachable within a realistic frame of time, most likely a year. If you are 60 lbs (27 kg) overweight, to use our previous example, it would be unrealistic to say you want to lose 60 lbs in a year. That would amount to losing 5lbs (2 kg), every single month of the year.

While this is possible the effort involved makes it unsustainable and it raises the possibility of injury, overtraining and maybe even metabolic shock, all of which in turn, make this target unrealistic.

What should you set then as your target goal? How about losing 24lbs, (10kgs), in that first year? That is only 2lbs, less than 1kg, a month for every month of the year. Still a hard target if we are talking about every single month of the year but definitely doable which then makes it more realistic. An even better plan would be to aim to lose 1.5lbs each month, about 0.6 kg, which makes it 18lbs (8kg), in the year. This way, should everything remain exactly the same which it won't, a 60lbs (27kg) weightloss becomes possible within a three year period.

If this tips you off about anything it is the fact that when it comes to fitness patience, which is a virtue, is an absolute necessity. Try to force anything too fast and you risk achieving the exact opposite. If you're looking to build strength and stamina you will end us overtraining and maybe, even, getting injured. If you try to lose weight your body's metabolism will change and make it harder to do so.

So patience is what you need to help you achieve your goals.

Unless you're a professional athlete with some very specific requirements, the ingredients of every fitness plan are more or less the same much the way the ingredients for cooking usually are protein, carbohydrates, fat and fiber. Yet, just as every meal we make is going to be a little bit different and reflect our particular needs, a little self-knowledge and perhaps even some awareness will go a long way towards formulating a fitness plan that can really deliver what we expect.

The fitness plan we shall put together will have three fundamental ingredients present. The proportions of each ingredient however will be different for each person because they depend on what each of us wants to achieve with this plan. Remember fitness is always personal and it is unique to us. What we do to meet the goals we have set ourselves reflects that uniqueness.

Fitness Plan Ingredients

- Strength
- Mobility
- Cardiovascular Fitness

Remember that this is a personal fitness plan designed to help you meet your fitness goals. If you're in your twenties and want to get fit to increase your appeal to potential romantic partners the mix of the ingredients in your fitness plan is going to be different than if you're in your fifties and want to be more active so you can keep up with your grandchildren.

The three ingredients mentioned here however are fundamental and, as we shall see in more detail in later chapters, they're key to building a body that stays functionally strong and healthy your entire life.

So, if you've thought long and hard about what kind of fitness goal you're aiming for and why you want it and have also managed to put together a decent workout program that will help you within the time you have postulated in your fitness plan, to get fitter and healthier then you're still not quite finished.

The execution phase of what you do also needs three key elements to come together so that your hard work shows results. These key elements are also fundamental and therefore non-negotiable. While the percentage of each in your fitness plan will vary according to your own personal circumstances, they all need to be present is some form for your plan to work.

Fitness Plan Execution

- Exercise
- Nutrition
- Sleep

The body only undergoes physical changes when it receives an adequately strong signal from its daily activities that it needs to change. We call this signal adaptation and it is the type of exercise we choose to engage in, its intensity and duration and frequency that actually provides it.

Adaptations however don't just happen. In order for them to take place the body needs to have the necessary resources to break down fat reserves for fuel to repair and build muscle. This is why good nutrition is so important. Finally, it's worth noting that the bulk of changes in the body and mind, only happen when we sleep. We only build muscle and repair tissue when our body can enjoy good quality sleep for approximately one third of the day.

Put Your Plan To Work

To make your plan work you need once again, three distinct parts that nonetheless, need to work seamlessly together:

- A goal that is realistic.
- A breakdown of the steps that'll get you to your goal.
- A way to measure the success you attain along the way to your goal.

Remember that the goal you set yourself is your direction. It's like a magnetic compass pointing North. Your North.

In our example of having an initial desire to lose 60lbs (27kg), in just twelve months, the most realistic goal we could set was to aim to lose 18lbs - (8 kg), over twelve months. That, in turn, breaks down to one and a half pounds of weight loss per month, which is just over half a kilogram. This amount of weightloss is realistic enough to achieve on average even if, for whatever reason, we fail to specifically hit that precise number a few times in the year.

To achieve this goal, realistic as it may be, the steps involved must also be thoroughly planned. Depending on how much available time you have, where you are and what equipment and space you have access to, you will need to work out a daily fitness routine that takes into account the fact that, on occasions, you will not feel like working out at all. This means that sometimes your workout intensity will be barely enough and there well also be times when you may not be able to workout at all for reasons beyond your immediate control. You will have to take all this into account.

To achieve the target that you set yourself you will need to factor in your 'good days' and 'bad days'. Good days are the days when working your plan goes like clockwork. Bad days are days when life throws a curve ball and all available time vanishes or days when everything, on a cumulative basis, simply gets too much and you just need a break.

What you have to do is create your plan in a way that allows you to realistically compensate for the 'bad days' so that when you do exercise on the 'good days' you don't have to overload your training to make up for lost ground.

How do you do that? Well, by simply putting in enough non-exercise activity thermogenesis (NEAT for short) in your everyday life. NEAT is a fancy term that stands for daily physical activity that isn't exercise. It uses slow-twitch muscles that use up a relatively small amount of energy when they're working but account for anywhere between 15 and 30 percent of daily energy expenditure. Some examples of NEAT activities are:

- Walk a minimum of 5,000 steps each day, every day.
- Take the stairs instead of the elevator, whenever you can.
- Do the ironing, mow the lawn, walk the dog or play ball with the kids.

There are many non-exercise activities that help us move our body and burn calories and they require no warm-up, no special planning, no special equipment nor indeed anything else beyond our ability to consciously create opportunities for them to happen, naturally every day.

By planning this way you will always be confident that no matter what setback you face as far as your formal exercise routine is concerned your plan is working because you are still maintaining a constant level of everyday activity in the background.

This makes it easier to reach the stated target from our example, of losing one and a half pounds of weight, per month.

The way we would measure success along the way, in this particular example is by simply stepping on the scales at the end of the month to see if that desired 1.5lbs (0.6 kg) weight has been lost and, perhaps checking halfway through the month to make sure that we're heading in the right direction and there are no surprises waiting for us ahead.

I used weightloss as an example because so many of us are preoccupied with it. Your fitness target can be anything, from an increase in muscle size to a change in body composition to an increase in endurance or speed. Regardless of what you aim to achieve the process will be the same and the methodology we employed here will always allow you to see how you're doing and what, if any, adjustments are necessary along the way.

It's important to keep a detailed written record of the structure of your plan, its execution and your progress otherwise you will run the risk of relying on how you feel you're doing in a particular moment which means you will either overestimate your achievements and risk losing momentum or be really harsh on yourself which will demoralize you, demotivate you and most likely make you stop.

Keeping a record of everything you do each day (and even the way you feel) is super-important if you are to achieve your stated goals. This then leads to one more and final for this chapter, three-step method you need to apply as you put your plan to work:

- Record
- Measure
- Analyze

Remember: you can never understand what you cannot record. You can never improve what you cannot measure. And, you can never control what you cannot analyze.

It doesn't matter if you use an app to keep track of everything digitally or an old-school method like keeping a paper journal. As long as you keep track of what you do and when you do it, you will always be able to understand how well you're doing.

Even more important is the fact that you will have this record when you are not doing well or when you're not getting the results you expect to get or when you find yourself stopping your fitness journey and then start again only to stop again and have to start all over again.

When you face so much friction every step of the way that getting your self mentally and physically fit feels like an uphill battle all the time, being able to go over the record of what you did and when; will help you identify what you can change and what you can do better.

Armed with all these steps then the only thing left to say in this chapter is that once you have your plan you need to work it. Have faith in the process and have faith in your self. Be persistent, be patient and above all be kind to your self.

Take Action

Problem: There is no "one size fits all" solution in fitness.

Solution: Define, for yourself, what fitness really means to you personally so you can make it work for you in the long term, without a significant amount of effort.

What To Do: Articulate, ideally in writing, how you see a fitter version of yourself in the very near future. Set a time frame not longer than twelve to eighteen months at the most. Be very detailed in your description.

Why: Articulate, ideally in writing again, the reasons that are important to you, which make you want to see this fitter version of yourself in the near future. Be honest. Be detailed. Be precise in describing your reasons and the emotions behind them that make those reasons important to you.

How: Detail, in writing, the general strategy you will employ to help you achieve this fitter version of yourself that you have visualized.

Action Plan

There are three steps to your action plan.

Step One: Set a goal. Check to see what it is that you articulated as your desired state of fitness in the time frame you've chosen. Determine what you will use as a measure of your progress. If, for example, your goal was to lose weight then, obviously, you will need to step on the scales at regular intervals to make sure you're heading in the right direction. If you're looking to build muscle and get stronger you will need to decide on the metric you will use to gauge the success of your efforts. The point is that without a metric which is truly reflective of your progress you will be unable to make any headway over the long term. Without a time frame that is reasonable you will set yourself up to fail because you will always feel you're under pressure to achieve.

Step Two: Put together a plan. Your plan is the execution. It is the practical steps you will take to meet your goal. It doesn't matter how well you may have visualized everything so far, if you fail to plan properly, you will fail. Here's how to avoid failing: In your plan take into account not just the practical steps you need to take every day in order to work out but also what you will do if unexpected situations occur that prevent you from working out. Your plan, in other words is not just the standard: I will walk for 40 minutes every day after lunch, variety. What happens if it's raining? What happens if your workload suddenly gets so much that you skip lunch? What happens if you need to travel out of town? What happens if you just had a crazy week and tiredness has caught up with you? Your plan, to work, needs to take all this into account, so it must have back-up plans in case your primary ones fail and your back-ups will need back-ups of their own. For instance, your 40-minute walk after lunch didn't happen. Fine. Can you find 5 minutes to do some step lunges and squats? No? How about 1 minute to do as many push-ups as you can in that time?

The examples used here are to guide you. Each time you face a challenge to your fitness plans it will be unique to you and your circumstances. If you plan for those eventualities however life may feel hectic and it may be messy but your fitness journey will always stay on track.

Step Three: Make everything easy. If in order to go and walk for 40 minutes after lunch you need to change shoes, find someone to mind the phone in the office, pick a path that's relatively clean and quiet, have some really nice weather and no massive workload to return to after you're done; you're setting yourself up to fail. The number of times all these will perfectly align in the year so you can keep yourself healthy will be very small indeed. If on the other hand the fitness activity you planned requires maybe one or, at the most, two steps like: Finish lunch, leave your office and walk outside for 40 minutes, then you're more likely to make it a regular thing, no matter what. The same easy-to-do logic applies to your back-up plans and the back-up to your back-up plans. Always choose activities that:

- Don't require a lot of thinking to make them happen.
- Are easy to access.
- You can do.

The workouts that follow are suggestions of structured physical activity you can engage in, though you are totally welcome to follow them exactly in the order they are presented. They cover a good range of capabilities and, to help you even further, a few exercise snacks have been thrown in that you could use as a back-up should your primary workout not happen for some reason.

There are eight DAREBEE workouts that follow. Each of these can be customized to your level by choosing to do Level I, II or III each of which has a different number of sets. You go from one illustrated exercise to the next in clockwise, left-to-right fashion. As per the instructions you take a rest of up to two minutes between sets. Most need no equipment and hardly any space. Pick the one you think best reflects your fitness level and capabilities and try to master it by doing it, eventually, to Level III.

AGAINST THE ODDS

DAREBEE WORKOUT © **darebee.com**

LEVEL I 3 sets **LEVEL II** 5 sets **LEVEL III** 7 sets **REST** up to 2 minutes

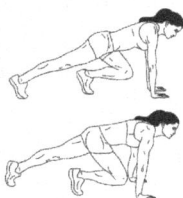

20 climbers

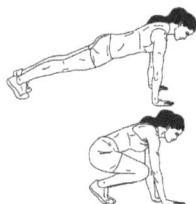

3 plank jump-ins

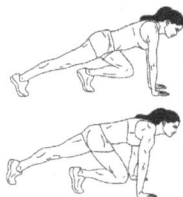

20 climbers

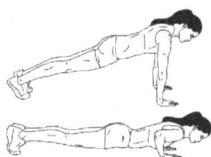

3 push-ups

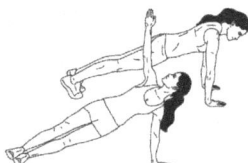

10 plank rotations

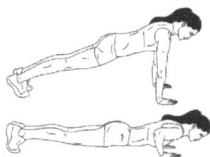

3 push-ups

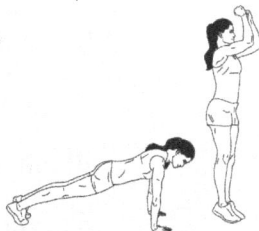

3 basic burpees

CARDIO BUNNY

DAREBEE WORKOUT © darebee.com
LEVEL I 3 sets **LEVEL II** 5 sets **LEVEL III** 7 sets
REST up to 2 minutes

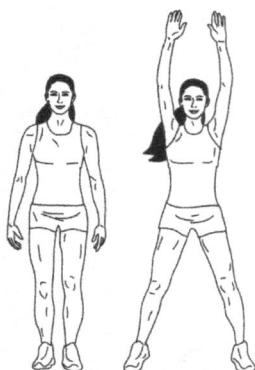

10 jumping jacks

3 squat hold hops

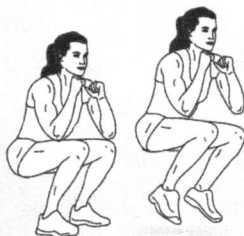

10 jumping jacks

3 squat hold hops

10 jumping jacks

3 squat hold hops

10 jumping jacks

3 squat hold hops

10 jumping jacks

3 squat hold hops

FULL-BODY
POWER

DAREBEE WORKOUT © darebee.com
LEVEL I 3 sets **LEVEL II** 4 sets **LEVEL III** 5 sets
REST up to 2 minutes

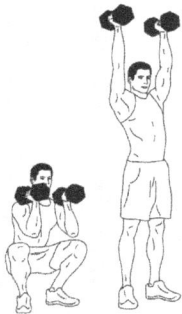

8 thrusters

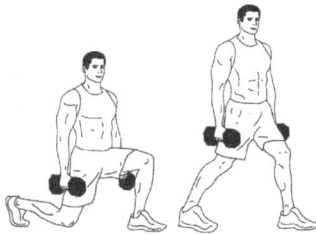

16 split lunges

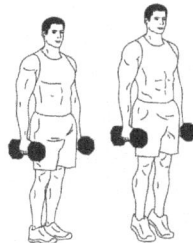

8 calf raises

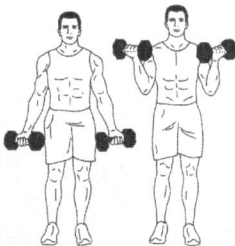

8 bicep curls

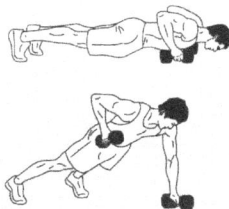

8 push-up renegade rows

clean break

DAREBEE WORKOUT © darebee.com

LEVEL I 3 sets **LEVEL II** 4 sets **LEVEL III** 5 sets **REST** up to 2 minutes

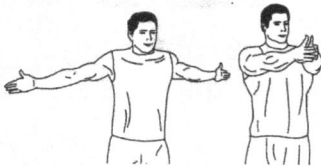

20 chest expansions

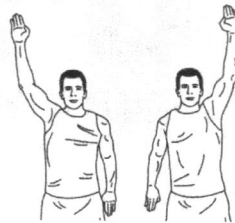

20 alt chest expansions

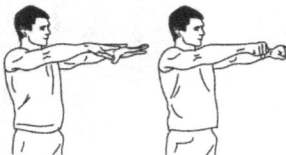

20 clench / unclench
arms forward

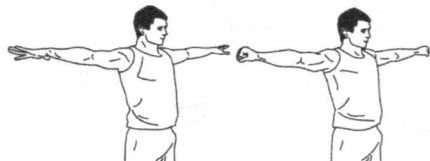

20 clench / unclench
arms to sides

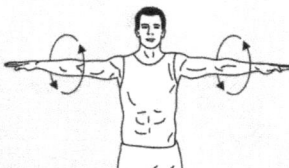

20 arm circles

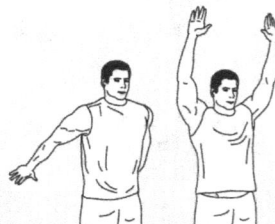

20 wide arm circles

cat girl

DAREBEE WORKOUT © darebee.com

LEVEL I 3 sets **LEVEL II** 4 sets **LEVEL III** 5 sets **REST** up to 2 minutes

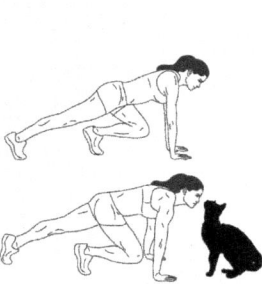

20 climbers

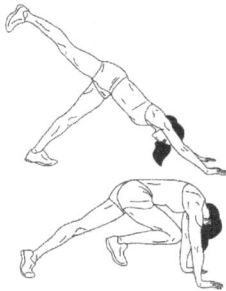

20 knee in & out

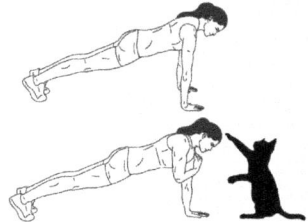

20 shoulder taps

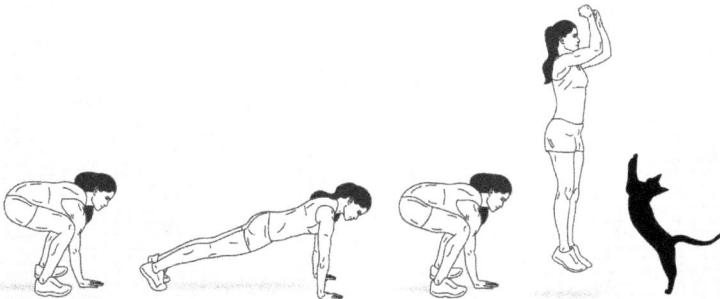

10 basic burpees

GUESS WHO IS BACK

DAREBEE WORKOUT
© darebee.com
60 seconds rest
between exercises

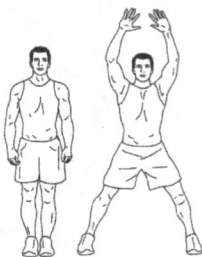

40 jumping jacks
5 sets | 60 seconds rest

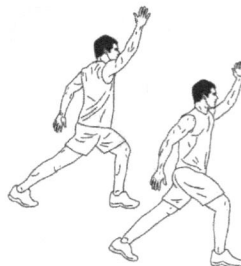

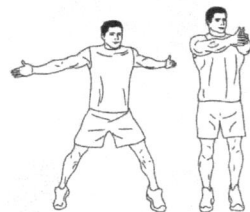

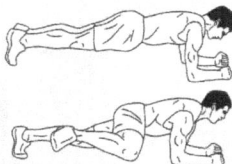

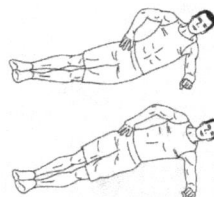

40 split jacks
5 sets | 60 seconds rest

40 seal jacks
5 sets | 60 seconds rest

20 elbow plank crunches
change sides and repeat
60 seconds rest

20 side bridges
change sides and repeat
60 seconds rest

DANCE PARTY
(IN MY KITCHEN)

DAREBEE WORKOUT © **darebee.com**

LEVEL I 3 sets **LEVEL II** 5 sets **LEVEL III** 7 sets **REST** up to 2 minutes

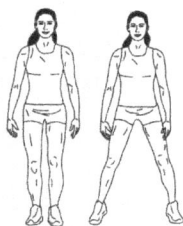

10 half jacks

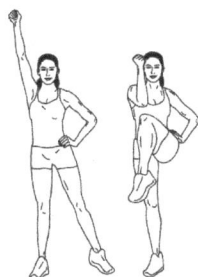

10 knee-to-elbow

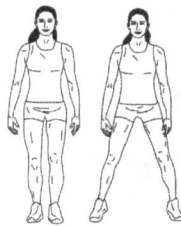

10 half jacks

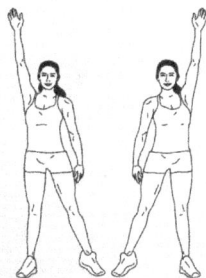

10 side jacks

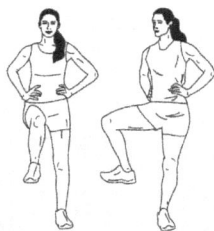

10 single hip rotations

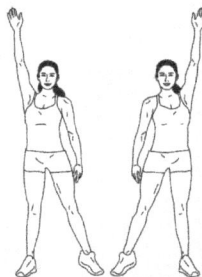

10 side jacks

UNBROKEN

DAREBEE WORKOUT © darebee.com

LEVEL I 3 sets **LEVEL II** 5 sets **LEVEL III** 7 sets **REST** up to 2 minutes

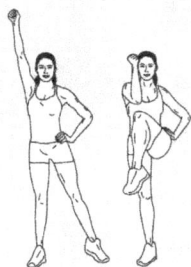

10 knee-to-elbow

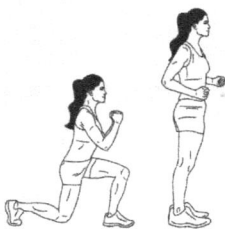

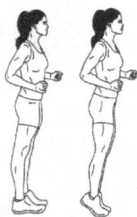

10 reverse lunges

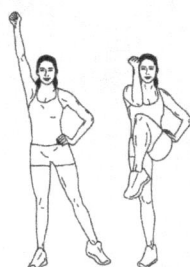

10 knee-to-elbow

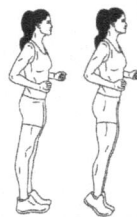

10 calf raises

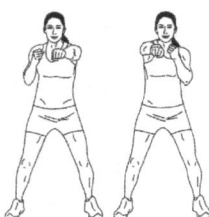

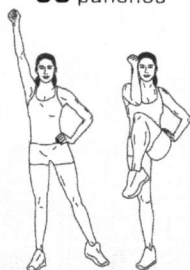

30 punches

10 calf raises

10 knee-to-elbow

The following four DAREBEE workouts are short. They're perfect to use as a back-up plan should you be unable to work out properly.

2-MINUTE ARMS

DAREBEE WORKOUT © darebee.com
20 seconds each exercise | no rest between exercises

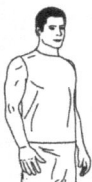

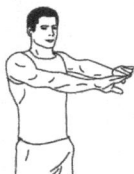

arm raises

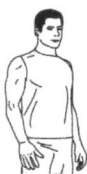

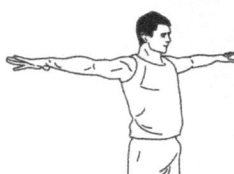

lateral arm raises

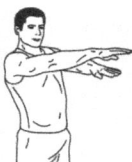

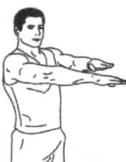

arm scissors

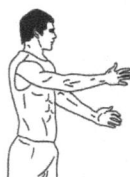

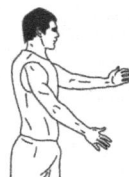

scissor chops

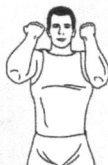

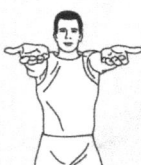

bicep extensions

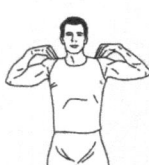

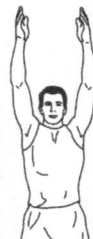

shoulder taps

HOLIDAY MODE

DAREBEE WORKOUT © darebee.com

EASY

60 seconds rest between exercises

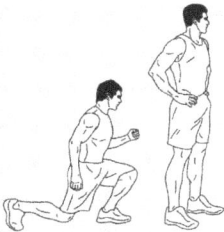

24 reverse lunges
3 sets | 30 seconds rest

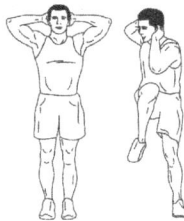

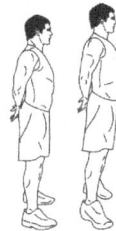

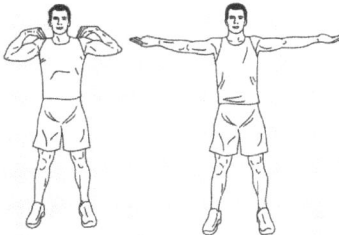

12 knee-to-elbow
3 sets | 30 seconds rest

12 calf raises
3 sets | 30 seconds rest

24 side shoulder taps
3 sets | 60 seconds rest

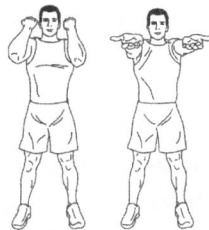

24 bicep extensions
3 sets | 60 seconds rest

WILLOW

DAREBEE WORKOUT © darebee.com

Hold each pose for 60 seconds then move on to the next one.

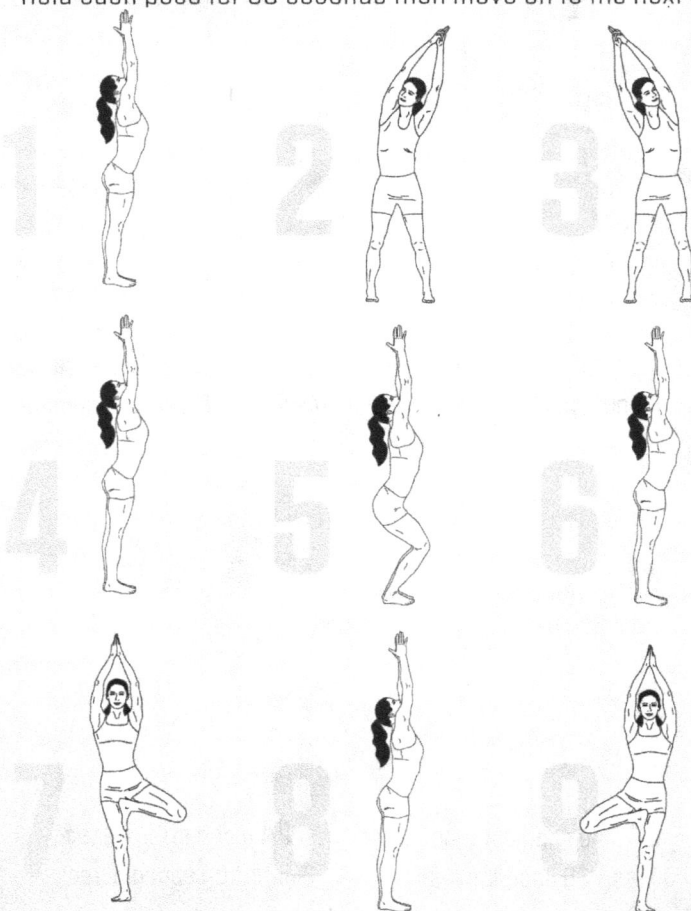

ALL THE
BASICS

DAREBEE
WORKOUT
© darebee.com
30 seconds rest
between exercises

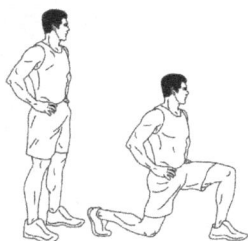

10 lunges
5 sets in total
30 second rest

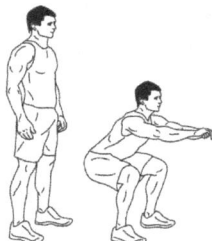

10 squats
5 sets in total
30 second rest

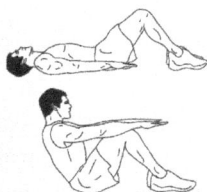

10 sit-ups
5 sets in total
30 second rest

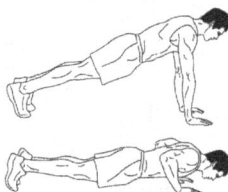

10 push-ups
5 sets in total
30 second rest

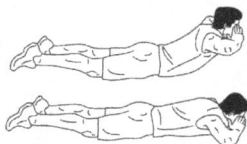

10 back extensions
5 sets in total
30 second rest

EMPOWERMENT AND CONTROL

We crave control in life long before we're in a position to reason or understand why things happen. Exercise is the one thing that can restore to us what we crave and yet we're programmed to avoid it.

If I were to ask you, right now: "What do you want to do?" What would be your answer?

This is a trick question. Logically, your reply depends on many factors: how well we know each other, where we're at, the time of day, the time of the month, our available cash (maybe), the subjects we usually talk about, what we were talking about just before I asked you that question. Your age. Your gender. Your family situation.

Context, it would appear, is everything here. And context defines us to such a degree that without it you and I and anyone else in our shoes would be unable to answer that simple question with any degree of seriousness or certainty.

Seriousness, as in meaningful intent, and certainty, in the sense that we know what's going on, are properties of context. A joke, a decision or an action that may be appropriate in one setting may be wildly inappropriate in a different one. Because context defines everything, every situation we find ourselves in is a little bit different from every other situation we've encountered before. When the degree of difference we sense gets past a threshold point that's defined by our own knowledge and experience we end up feeling unprepared for the situation we find ourselves in.

Being unprepared means we may not feel able to judge a situation correctly or know exactly how we should behave so that we don't make a fool of ourselves and we don't suffer any material or reputational damage.

Inevitably the level of stress we experience in such situations rises, as it should, because the stress response is there to help us become more alert and energized. What allows us to navigate these uncharted situations better and manage the stress response so it does not overwhelm us is the sense of empowerment and control we have over ourselves and over our life.

We shall get to the scientific definition of both empowerment and control a little later in this chapter but first I will illustrate the practical aspects of both through a real life story.

And this real life story starts with a 12 year old boy living in the 1970s who finds himself in Queensland, Australia, having moved there with his family, from New South Wales. He is in a new school, a new state, a new city and an entirely different culture.

Although that boy has not got a bad home life he does not have adequate parental supervision or support as he tries to navigate all this. Inevitably he feels stressed, alienated, alone. This becomes even more so given the fact that at 12 he is also balancing at the cusp of becoming a young adult and being no longer a child.

That young boy, had he been in our time, would have reached perhaps for Playstation and lost himself in the world of gaming or got into online apps and social media. But being the 70s that is not really an option.

There are drugs of course but they're hard to find and they cost money and that 12-year-old boy hasn't got ready access to money (or people who sell drugs). There is alcohol but that too is a little out of reach as there are strict state alcohol laws that require an ID as proof of age.

Watching TV is not an option either as TV hours are weird in the 70s (TV stations stop broadcasting after midnight during the week) and daytime TV content, when it is available, is geared to a stay-at-home older audience. Playing what video games are available in the 1970s (alongside pinball machines) is limited to arcades and it is expensive so the option is not really one that can work for him long term.

Luckily for him, perhaps, that young boy reads comic books and the Marvel and DC universes provide a ready means of escape that help him decompress a little. But even this means of escape is limited. While the cost of a comic book is easily within that boy's purchasing power he still has to wait every week for a comic book in the series he follows to come out on a specific day of the week. Being dependent on the publishing schedules of comic book publishers and the delivery times of local news agents is hardly conducive to creating any sense of empowerment or control.

Comic books do something else. Beyond providing a means of escape and a great way to explore complex moral issues, they also provide a strong, visually appealing aesthetic of athleticism that this boy is enamored by.

His comic book heroes, despite their superpowers, seem to struggle with the same complex social issues of not fitting in, isolation and alienation that he does. And they channel some of that angst they feel into physical action. They run and jump and cavort on the comic book page. They hit punch bags and practice shadow boxing.

And it is this that leads that young boy growing up in the 1970s, a world that seems in retrospect almost entirely alien to us today, to take up running. He starts by getting up in the morning before he goes to school to run around the block on his own.

He discovers that running provides a release that lasts long afterwards. Because this is Brisbane, Australia in the 1970s and there really is not much else to do, everybody plays sport. Being fit provides the boy with an easy way to either stand out or blend in, depending on the situation.

His morning runs become longer. He finds himself cutting into his sleep time to get more running time in. And he starts training at home on his own, doing push-ups and sit-ups in his bedroom. And because all this helps him channel the inner turmoil he feels, he takes the next step in his athletic journey and on his 13th birthday he joins a martial arts club to learn Karate.

What he discovers is that the intense training he does at the martial arts club and the extra work he puts in at home and before school allow him to feel at peace with himself throughout his day. This leads to a change in behavior. He focuses more in class. He learns to revel in the feeling of understanding things using his brain. Because he uses physical action to escape and decompress, to feel empowered and in control of his life, he can then turn to study as an additional form of escape that also gives him an added sense of empowerment and control.

There is a cascade of changes that take place for that boy, both inside and out. Because he studies more he becomes academically accomplished. He becomes an A-grade student. Because he exercises he takes part in every school sport activity he can, becoming a star athlete. And because he both exercises and studies, he has the necessary clarity of mind to understand that just like physical training allows him to escape the inner turmoil and angst he feels, academic training will enable him to escape from the then rural and restrictive surroundings of his home town.

In due course he is at University studying Chemical Engineering. He doesn't know it yet but his knowledge and understanding of physical and chemical processes and mathematics will allow him to turn what he knows into an international career that will see him, as an adult, criss-cross the globe working with executives of Fortune 100 companies around the world. He will write books on marketing and pen the first popular book on semantic search and be invited to speak at conventions in places as diverse from each other as New York city and Las Vegas or Singapore and Shanghai.

That young boy is me. Without really planning to, led only by circumstances and the choices available to me I discovered, entirely by accident, the power of exercise to help me control my emotional states. Long before neuroscience was a globally accepted field of study capable of revealing the innermost secrets of the brain and body, I'd discovered; entirely by chance the equation that says: Motion = Emotion.

When you really think about it this is not so novel. We frequently say "jump for joy" expressing the concept that intense, inner feelings are made visible through movement. This is universal human behavior that is observable across times and cultures as an expression of emotion.

Through what hindsight will label a serendipitous chain of events I managed to mediate the insidious and dangerous discomfort of emotional isolation and social alienation by embracing the discomfort of exercise which gave me a feeling of empowerment and control over my life.

Subconsciously this established a pattern of behavior that, again without planning or even a lot of thinking, persisted throughout my entire adult life. By my 18th birthday I was a Black Belt in Wado Ryu. By the time I was 22 I had a Black Belt in WTF Tae Kwon Do and by the time I was 25 I had a Black Belt in ITF Tae Kwon Do and was taking part in national competitions in Britain.

By 27 I had a 2nd degree Black Belt in ITF Tae Kwon Do and was officially a certified Tae Kwon Do instructor.

In the 15 year space between the 12-year-old me and my 27-year-old self I had moved countries three times and was living in an entirely different continent. I had a romantic partner, a mortgage and a high-powered job that demanded 50 contact hours a week. And I still got up at 6.00 am to run before work and I still managed to train intensively for two hours every evening.

Outsiders looking in will say that's "discipline". They will tell you this is "dedication". They will point out that in fitness you need to have discipline and dedication to get results. From the outside in they're right. People who repeatedly and persistently engage in high-level physical activity look strong and appear healthy. Only half of this is true.

Was my then self, strong and fast and fit? Without a doubt. I was training seven days a week, 52 weeks a year, holding down a high-powered career and working long hours five days a week and I appeared to be able to do all this with ease. But was I truly healthy? Was my internal world at peace? Was I mentally serene? Were my everyday responses to stimuli balanced? Was I stress-free?

The only person qualified to answer that is me. With the power of hindsight I can see that what helped keep my mind this side of sanity, barely, was the fact that I was using exercise as a self-administered medication. It was my one and only coping mechanism.

I needed exercise to help me deal with the challenges in my life and I embraced it wholeheartedly because the only time I felt serene and collected was when I pushed myself to the limits of my physical ability. That's the only time my head truly cleared and it was a feeling of clarity and peace that lasted with me a few hours afterwards.

The point this true story drives home is that a simple accident of circumstances helped me find a viable way to control my life in a way that happened to also benefit me in the long term.

Life is chaotic for everyone. The degree may differ but we all experience forces we cannot control which then make us react to circumstances we have not created. This makes us feel stressed and helpless and when we feel stressed and helpless our body produces cortisol which is a stress hormone that impacts the liver, muscle, adipose tissue, and pancreas. When in the liver, "high cortisol levels increase gluconeogenesis and decrease glycogen synthesis." As a result we put on weight, feel weaker and become unhealthier.

The more uncomfortable we feel in our body the more unhealthy and weak that body becomes. Our behavior is the result of our internal states and when those internal states are unbalanced our behavior also appears off. We may become intolerant. We may anger easily. We may overreact to situations. We may feel overwhelmed. We may be incapable of clear thinking. If we exhibit any or all of these symptoms, it is a sign that inside our skin and behind our eyes we experience stress and discomfort we cannot articulate and have no means of mitigating.

Left unchecked, without intervention, that process takes us down a catastrophic spiral where we feel less and less in control of the one thing we should, by rights, be able to control at will: our own physical body. If we cannot feel in control of our body it becomes virtually impossible to achieve control and mastery of our life.

We become locked in thoughts, choices, actions and behaviors that fail to give us the positive outcomes we seek and consign us to lash out every time things become too much. This is where "empowerment" and "control" come in.

The scientific definition of empowerment is that it is a process which enables each person to understand the relationship between what they do and the results they achieve. This better understanding of the connection between actions and outcomes allows us to create the power to achieve the results we desire in our life by planning what we do so that we can achieve what we want.

The scientific definition of control is the perception an individual has of their power to affect their circumstances, environment and their own emotional states. On that last item, in particular, psychology states that what separates us from the other animals around us is our ability to manage our impulses, emotions, and behaviors to achieve long-term goals.

If we were to go back, right now, to that opening sentence of this chapter and I were to ask you "what do you want to do?" how much of your answer now would be informed by your own better understanding of the empowerment and control you have in your own life? What has hopefully changed between the moment I initially posed this question to you and right now is that your understanding of the context of your life has, hopefully, broadened.

You can now see a little more clearly, I hope, the things you do control and the things you don't and the things you want to control. You can see a little more clearly what you are truly capable of and how your own thoughts lead to choices that lead to actions which have an effect. The cumulative effect of these actions is your life.

Exercise is a Stressor

If we only did things that are good for us in the long term you wouldn't be reading this book right now because you wouldn't need it. Notice how I used a qualifier: long term.

No one knowingly acts to hurt themselves. This includes every conceivable human activity in every conceivable scenario you care to come up with. Smoking, drinking, eating too much of all the wrong foods, beating ourselves up mentally, beating ourselves up physically, taking drugs. Whatever form of self-harm or potential self-harm you care to mention you can bet that there is a corpus of scientific evidence which shows that it provides a temporary form of release from an otherwise toxic or unbearable situation we find ourselves in.

Even suicide, the ultimate form of self-harm, is at the moment of ideation and even its action, a release from a situation that creates an increase in feelings of depression, stress and anxiety. These feelings are represented by neurochemical changes that unbalance our internal state and create a certain amount of neurochemically-induced toxicity which, in turn, makes us feel so unbearably bad that the crazy idea of taking our own life can seem like a reasonable avenue of escape.

What this suggests is that life is full of stressors and we are so hardwired to seek to avoid stressors that we engage in adaptive responses. Some of those adaptive responses can compromise our long-term longevity and undermine our long-term health.

If we can so easily engage in what essentially are acts of self-harm logic suggests that we should also be able to engage with at least the same level of ease in acts, like exercise, that are beneficial to us.

We don't.

Here's why: exercise is a stressor.

No one really is going to ever tell you this to your face. Everywhere you look: ads on TV and in glossy magazines and videos on the internet show you happy, smiling people fully engaged in physical activity with a broad grin on their face.

Ads are not reality. Not even close. And everyone you see is selling you something: clothes, shoes, equipment, membership, supplements or a location.

Exercise is a physical and mental stressor and we are hardwired to avoid stressors which means that paradoxically, we're hardwired to avoid the very same type of physical activity we need to keep us healthy and help us live longer.

Because we are not entirely irrational beings we may convince ourselves, as the year ends and we take stock of where we have been and where we need to go, to get a gym membership or start a gym class on the other side of Christmas.

Gyms across the United States report a membership increase of up to 13% on the 1st day of January but by mid-February most of those people have stopped and by March nearly all of them have. The figures are surprisingly similar in Britain where lifestyles, culture and the weather are different.

The issue is not so much culture or expectations or advertising as it is human behavior which is depressingly similar everywhere and, as a result, dispiritingly predictive.

And it is human behavior that guides us to fail at our most cherished and most popular New Year's resolution each year.

To our credit the most popular New Year resolutions have to do with us getting healthier because, I suppose, as we consciously realize an entire year has gone by and another one is about to begin we become more conscious of time and aging and we then want to do something proactive and meaningful which will help us stave off the inevitability of old age, decrepitude and death.

We are not stupid. Nor are we in denial. The passage of time, we understand, is unstoppable. We all understand that when it comes to how we feel and the quality of life we can enjoy; we can do better.

And we are right.

So, so far so good. But the figures are depressing. According to a U.S. gym owners' survey by May each year, eight out of ten people will have dropped out citing a variety of reasons. Those who don't drop out will exercise less than four hours a week which is definitely better than dropping out and doing nothing but nowhere near enough to achieve what they need.

Why does this happen? The answer, again, is because exercise is a stressor and we are hardwired to avoid stressors. I cannot repeat this enough. Paradoxically activities which harm us, are also stressors. We only need to look at the cascade of neurochemical events that take place in the body if we smoke just one cigarette, to understand that. But unlike exercise the activities which harm us do not appear to be stressors. Smoking a cigarette will not tire us out, make us sweat, drain our body of energy or leave us out of breath. Drinking alcohol doesn't feel like self-harm. Neither does overeating.

In contrast in the ancient past where our bodies were forged the physical activity that today we call exercise: the running and the sprinting, the jumping and the kicking, the lifting and the throwing was physical activity we undertook as an essential aspect of our daily life.

We all did all that without question because our mind was focused on our need to survive. We needed to run and to jump and to lift and to throw. Sometimes we even needed to fight in order to survive. And when we didn't have to do any of that our ancient body, very cleverly, developed a predisposition that made us want to sit around a campfire and talk and have fun and eat and then go to sleep.

These were things that made us happy because our everyday physical life was full of stressors we could not avoid and the only way we could successfully navigate it was to grab enough rest so we could recover and be in a position to do all those things all over again the next day.

What we today call being lazy is a natural response to experienced stress that was intended to help us survive.

No wonder then that New Year's fitness resolutions are not kept and no wonder we find exercising sufficiently to get fit, a difficult thing to do, willingly, for long. We are not really designed to seek it out.

There are exceptions of course and they prove the rule. My particular story case in point. Because the stress I experienced growing up, on a daily basis, was high I adopted the stressor of exercise as my escape route. In the process I taught myself to embrace it, embrace the discomfort and the pain because that took my mind away from the deeper and more persistent problems I was facing.

Athletes who go on to compete at the highest level in their sport have also managed to flip this switch in their head in the exact same way. They embrace the pain and the sacrifice involved in pursuing their chosen discipline because it provides them with the route necessary to escape the particular pressures of their life. By actively choosing to subject themselves to a stressor they do control they achieve a measure of empowerment and control that the other circumstances in their life deny them. As a result they function much better in the world.

That, certainly, was my case. It did not matter to me how much discomfort I felt while exercising or how sore my body was the next day. Those were things I had chosen for myself and because I had chosen to subject myself to that experience I felt empowered by my ability to make that choice and be in control of my own life.

The logical question to ask here then is: if exercise as a stressor has such amazing benefits and it can provide us with a readily available means to escape the helplessness of life, one that is side-effects free and relatively low cost, why isn't it already something that everyone chooses to do?

It is a great question and one whose answer lies two inescapable and interlinked elements one is the relatively slow speed at which see the effects of exercise. The other is a mental calculus we all engage in that behavioral scientists call "temporal discounting" whose net effect is to reduce our sense of the value of a likely reward when that reward lies in the future and is also uncertain.

To illustrate this point ask yourself which sounds best to you: "Get a Beach Body in just four weeks" or "Live a long and healthy life through a lifelong commitment to our highly structured exercise and diet plan"?

The example is carefully weighted of course to produce the response I want from you but then so is every ad you see for diets, fitness and even health.

The truth is that of all the stressors available to us to employ as countermeasures that mitigate any internal anxiety and stress we feel as a result of living in this world, exercise is the one that produces the slowest and maybe most uncertain results.

Every benefit exercise produces is the result of changes that are triggered by the experience of cumulative stress over time. Clarity of mind, emotional regulation, situational awareness, physical fitness, endurance, internal states stability - all of these happen gradually. And they happen only if we continue to exercise. And to happen in the best way possible with the most desirable results we must also manage our food intake and sleep time properly.

The variables pile on and the uncertainty increases which is why we become, for lack of a better term, "exercise shy".

Yet the benefits of exercise, as a whole, are undeniable. They are usually the direct result of the physical and mental stress induced by exercise itself. Some of them, like the relief from psychological or mental stress are fairly immediate. We all feel psychologically freer and mentally clearer after a good, hard run. But we have to be able to run long enough and hard enough for that to happen. And that means we have to already be sufficiently fit to do that.

If we're not fit enough already to choose a long, hard run as our avenue of escape, trying to run long enough and hard enough is such a hard physical and mental stressor that it is likely to make us, after a first attempt, to never want to do it again.

This is the problem in a nutshell then: exercise can help us feel stronger and be healthier but exercise is difficult and we are programmed to avoid anything labeled 'difficult'. So unless we are already strong enough for physical activity to be one of the tools in our arsenal for decompression from the pressures of life, choosing it only adds to our problems, at first and solves nothing in the short term.

When we see exercise from this perspective it's no wonder so few people exercise. Certainly I wouldn't. Neither would you. The good news is that there is a way to get round this problem. Knowing that it occurs for our own good because of our body's ancient responses which however no longer serve us well in a modern setting, we can use our smart brains to get what we want.

Before I give you the formula for this I will explain how I found the solution to this problem almost by accident.

Understand The Stressor Avoidance Response

I have already explained how, because of my personal circumstances, I stumbled upon exercise as an interventionary measure to help me manage the stress of my daily life. We have already seen why we tend to avoid exercise and, within the ancient evolutionary logic of our body and brain, this avoidance makes perfect sense.

What we need now is to find a way to make our body want to exercise. Because we no longer live in a world that is physically hostile to us we have to find a way to circumvent the ancient imperatives that stop us from doing what we know will be good for us in the long term.

As I am writing this I am a few weeks shy from my 60th birthday and by the time you read it I will be well past it. I still exercise every day. I still push myself to develop better physical skills and maintain the ones I already have. But the journey has been anything but smooth.

I stopped doing martial arts competitions in 2000. I was 35 and it was the turn of the century and I used that symbolic moment to transition to a life that focused a little more on career and a little more on personal development.

What I didn't know when I made that decision was the massive amount of difficulty I would run into the moment I stopped competing.

Martial arts competitions created, for me, an artificial environment that provided me with a sense of purpose. I'd get up at 6.00am every day and run 5km before work no matter what the weather was doing outside. I'd come home at 6.30pm and go training every evening for two hours. And I would do that five days a week and then train on my own or with friends on the weekends. All year round.

Crazy as that schedule was it served a distinct purpose which I would not really discover for over a decade later: it gave me a sense of empowerment over my life and a sense of control over who I was.

The moment I stopped competing however all that stopped too. Virtually overnight I went from putting in 16-17 hours of training a week to barely making three.

Worse than that, on those days when I did exercise, I found it harder and harder to push myself. As a result I started losing ground. Slowly, but surely. First I became a little slower. I was no longer as fast in my sprinting or punching or kicking. Then, I became a little heavier. A couple of extra kilograms (approximately five pounds). Again, nothing that was readily noticeable but still something that was there. And I started to lose my stamina. A 5km run became harder to do. A one-hour training session three times a week suddenly felt like a lot.

For the first time in my life I started to drink alcohol. Occasionally, but I did. You see life did not stop placing pressures on me just because I decided to stop competing and focus on my career more. Quite the opposite in fact. And though I was no longer that super stressed-out teen who discovered exercise as an avenue of escape there were still pressures that piled on me: a mortgage, bills, career, life stuff, marriage, divorce - in short, the things that pile on everyone of us and some that only pile on some of us, and somehow I still needed to find ways to decompress.

Whenever I took stock of myself mentally I would see that my fitness had slipped. In the years between the age of 35 when I stopped competing in martial arts and 45 when I finally found the clarity inside my head that I needed, I understood that I had to shape up but I found it difficult to do so and my brain gave me a lot of smart excuses to not do so: "I can get back into shape any time", I would tell myself. "I am in pretty good physical condition for someone my age," I would say at other times. "I no longer do martial arts competitions, I don't need to be that fit", I would think.

All of this was true. None of it served any other purpose than to let me off the hook so that I wouldn't have to do something about my lack of commitment to my fitness and long term health.

Beyond the fact that I no longer had an immediate, pressing target to aim for: i.e. martial arts competitions, I was also battling against two other adverse mechanisms that I was unaware of at the time and therefore didn't know how to handle.

The two silent enemies that I was fighting which I didn't even know existed back then and which hold you back too when you think about your fitness neuroscientists and psychologists today describe as: "temporal discounting" which we have already talked about a little, and "present bias".

We will take a detailed look at each because their scientific definition explains their devastating ability to undermine our efforts to improve physically.

Two Hidden Enemies

Behavioral science defines temporal discounting as "the process by which a reward loses value as a function of the delay to its receipt". In other words the longer the gap between an action we undertake and the moment we receive our reward for that action the more we are inclined to reduce the value that action represents for us.

Exercise is the perfect example. We exercise in the here and now. The rewards of that action however are in the future. No matter how hard we exercise in the present or for how long, we will not see any real benefits for weeks, months or even years in the future, depending of course on what we are aiming for.

If we want to get stronger and lift weights it will take at least eight weeks before we start to see any measurable results. If we want to improve our stamina it will take anywhere from eight to twelve weeks before we can begin to feel that we can exercise harder or run longer without feeling tired.

If we want to lose weight, depending on where we are at with our current weight and its deviation from our ideal weight it can take years before we begin to truly see the results we seek.

As if temporal discounting was not bad enough on its own, when it comes to exercise it combines really easily with that other psychological phenomenon called present bias. Present bias is the tendency we all experience in a trade-off situation to go for the smaller, immediate reward rather than wait for a larger and probably uncertain one in the future.

To understand how that works consider that were we to be presented with a chocolate bar right now we'd all immediately know exactly how amazing it will taste and how nice I will feel if we just ate it. But if we chose not to eat it we'd have no idea whether it will truly contribute to our losing weight at some point in the future, for example. The variables between this moment right now where we all want to just eat the chocolate bar, and the moment in the future where we experience some health benefit because we have put off eating it are too many to calculate with any degree of accuracy. It is the tangible, immediate and certain effect of eating the chocolate bar that makes it so hard to resist.

Present bias trips us up in many different and very cunning ways: we say it's too cold to go for a run. We explain to our self how today we had a hectic day and are just too tired to even attempt to exercise. We provide ourselves with countless excuses that sound factual, reasonable and are based on how we feel the moment we say them. They are backed up by an almost tangible extrapolation of the immediate reward we receive (i.e. relieved to not get cold or tired or physically exhausted etc) if we just don't exercise this instant which is why we, usually, end up not exercising.

This is a mode of thought that traps us in a downward spiral. By not exercising we become physically weaker so exercise becomes even more of an immediate stressor which we are hardwired to avoid so we end up doing even less and when we do force ourselves to exercise we feel bad anyway and that only reinforces the aversion we feel each time we think about exercising when we are busy, stressed, distracted, anxious or tired.

By now you are beginning, I hope, to see a solution of sorts: if our brain is hardwired for us to avoid exercise because exercise is a stressor and we are programmed by evolution to avoid stressors then we have to find a way to rewire that response so that we can do what will help us live a long, healthy and hopefully happy life.

For me it happened organically as, I suspect, it happens for a lot of top-flight amateur athletes who willingly put their bodies under immense stress day after day as they pursue excellence in their chosen sport.

Luckily for you, you don't have to work hard to work out how to do it for yourself because there is a relatively simple formula and a methodology you can apply that will help you rewire your brain so that it no longer trips you up so easily.

Rewiring The Stressor Avoidance Response

Intuitively we understand that exercise gives us the power to remake our body. If we lift weights we become strong. If we sprint we become fast. If we run long we become more durable. Each of these changes involves a host of physical and neurological adaptations that must take place. We rewire the way our body moves and functions by growing more muscles and then growing more nerves that control those muscles. We then have to produce more blood vessels and capillaries to feed those muscles. And we learn to control the extra muscles we have built through the new nerves we grow.

All of it is powered by adenosine triphosphate (ATP for short) which is produced and replenished from glucose. While the body has three sources of fuel, in truth it only uses ATP and everything else, through a complex cycle that depends on the physical activity we engage in, its intensity and duration, basically uses up carbohydrates, and glucose is a form of carbohydrates, to do keep us physically active.

Some of the changes triggered by exercise, like our ability to do something better or faster become plain to see. Bigger and better defined muscles are also obvious to the naked eye. What we don't see are the changes that happen in our brain. The brain is like any other organ in our body. It is supplied with nutrients through a network of blood vessels and it is wired with nerves. Unlike any other organ in our body however its work remains largely unseen.

If we run our heart beats faster and we can actually feel that. If we place our hand over the center of our chest and a little to the left, we get to directly experience the heart beating hard. If we lift heavy weights our arms get tired and we totally feel the work the muscles do. If we run fast for a long time we eventually get out of breath and we can feel our lungs working hard to re-oxygenate our bloodstream.

Yet, we never feel our brain working. We may think with it and be aware that we think with it but it just cannot actually feel it doing any visible work at all. At just over two per cent of the average bodyweight the brain accounts for nearly 20%, which is one fifth, of our daily energy needs. When something so relatively small requires so much of our daily energy to function, it stands to reason that it does both complex and important work. But we don't have a sense of that. Our brain doesn't get delayed onset muscle soreness (the so called DOMS) after we read a difficult book or watch a complex movie.

Our muscles do, even our lungs can feel bruised the day after a really hard cardiovascular session. But our brain feels like it does nothing strenuous.

The reason for this discrepancy in how we perceive our brain lies in the fact that the brain has no nociceptors. Nociceptors are the nerve endings that send signals to the brain from every part of the body. The pressure we feel when we accidentally bump our shoulder against a wall, which is interpreted as pain comes from the nociceptors. The brain has none. Without nociceptors to send signals the brain's discomfort at being stressed goes unacknowledged. We therefore feel like it does no work, feels no strain and can sustain no damage as a result. None of this is true except the nociceptor part.

The brain, just like any other organ in the body works incredibly hard, it can strain itself and get tired and it can sustain damage. Just like any other organ in the body the brain can be made to change.

Just like any other organ in the body the changes the brain makes are a direct, adaptive response to sustained environmental pressures it encounters. This adaptive response is fundamental in our physical make up. Of all the animals on the planet we are by far the most adaptive and by far the one most capable of remaking ourselves both inside and out.

We no longer live in caves or on trees in the wild. The environmental pressures we are exposed to are mostly man-made ones and the stresses we are subjected to are mostly man-made ones too. Getting our brain to adapt and change and rewire itself in the way we want it to requires three things:

- An awareness of what it is we are trying to do.
- A recognition of our eventual aim.
- A clear understanding of the process and path required to get us there.

This three-step approach is key to achieving desirable, lasting rewiring of the brain which results in the behavioral changes we want to see in our self.

Three Steps To A New Brain

The process for rewiring the brain is the same regardless of what it is we are trying to achieve. It can be applied equally well to something as intellectual as getting to like reading so that you read more books every year or something as practical as learning to be more patient with a relative so that you can have harmonious relations with them.

In our case we want to use it to make our brain stop avoiding exercise. Because the brain has no nociceptors that can signal pain and discomfort we will have to use feelings and emotions as our guide because we are aware of them.

Our reluctance to exercise manifests itself in a variety of feelings. A tightness in the chest and the pit of our stomach that make us feel tense when we consider the time has come to exercise. A sudden awareness of pains, aches and fatigue in our body that make us reluctant to want to engage in anything that is going to be physically demanding. A sense of overall malaise which we usually interpret as "not being in the mood" or "not feeling it".

Here's a truth no one usually discusses: no matter how fit you are. No matter how hard you have taught yourself to train and no matter how much physical exercise means to you, these feelings will persist. To a varying degree they will appear every time you consider exercise. I call these "pre-exercise nerves" and they hardly ever go away.

When exercise becomes a habit what becomes better, over time, is our ability to understand the source of the feelings that undermine our willingness to exercise and the reason they arise. This awareness then allows us to deal with them better so they do not derail what we are trying to achieve.

If these feelings never go away, you will now ask, is there any real point to trying to rewire the brain so that it handles the stressor of exercise better and you get to exercise more? The answer is: absolutely!

Make no mistake. Exercise will always be a perceived stressor. These nagging, niggling feelings at the back of your mind will always be there. But the moment you successfully rewire your brain you gain the instant capacity to better deal with the perceived stressor called exercise and to better handle the nagging, niggling feelings associated with pre-exercise nerves.

How do you go about this rewiring in practical terms? Here are the three key steps to help you do so:

* Awareness
* Recognition
* Understanding

Let's unpack each one in turn.

First step, Awareness: We have to start with an awareness of what it is we want to achieve in concrete, measurable terms. This is important. We cannot change something we cannot measure. And we cannot control anything that we cannot change. So if we say to ourselves, as an example, "I want to get fitter" the word fitter has to have a measurable change. If fitter means sprinting faster than we need to know our sprint time and have a realistic target to achieve that would help us measure improvement. If fitter means lifting more, or running longer, again we need to establish our starting baseline and then set our first, intermediate goal that will show that we are improving at what we do. If, for example, our personal best sprint for 100m is 20 seconds, we cannot expect to realistically drop it down to half that time in six months or even a year. But we can realistically aim for 19 seconds in six months and maybe an incremental improvement of one or two more seconds over the course of a year.

I mention sprinting specifically because it makes such physical demands of us that it is a multi-modal physical activity. You can substitute sprinting with any physical activity you engage in, provided you can break down the measurement of your anticipated improvement into reasonable steps.

Awareness then is the articulation of our specific fitness goals in a way that is reasonable and in a way that is measurable. This is the first step.

Second step, Recognition: We need to recognize what the end goal is for us. This second step may change over time as your age and circumstances also change, but it is always a key requirement. What is the end game? When I was doing martial arts competitions the end game for me was winning. That was it. Because winning in my mind required that I do everything that was physically possible in my training, I was willing to overlook any degree of physical discomfort and accept the grueling demands of daily training all year round so I could hit my target.

You will be different because each one of us is different in our aspirations and ambitions. What will be the same for you as it was for me however is the need to articulate that end game. It could be losing 30lbs as an example. Or being able to play with your grandchildren, or just feeling good inside your skin regardless of your age and gender. You will find it easy to recognize your end goal because it directly contributes to your feeling of empowerment and control in your life.

Remember you need to achieve empowerment and control over your life in order to reduce the levels of stress you experience. You need a sense of empowerment and control to help you build the resilience you need to successfully deal with unexpected events and unforeseen stressors.

The ability to do this causes fewer instances of prolonged and damaging internal states and helps us maintain our longterm health.

The moment you identify what it is you need in order to have the sense of empowerment and control over your life that you crave, you will have recognition of your end goal.

We're now ready for the third step: Understanding. If we are aware of what it is we need to achieve in order to have a sense of improvement in ourselves and we have recognized what the end goal is for us, we now need to understand in practical terms the daily actions we must engage in order to achieve all this.

Understanding is all about practicalities. Understanding is about the plan we put together that will enable us to get to our end goal. If awareness is the game and recognition is the strategy then understanding is the coach.

We need to have that understanding in order to be able to engage in the specific daily physical activity we need to achieve our end goal.

The end goal for me was winning martial arts competitions. To achieve that I ran 5km every day whatever the weather, did more than three hours of stretching a week and trained in a competitive martial arts club environment for two hours every night.

If your end goal is, as an example, to get strong enough by the end of the year to be able to lift your grandchild in the air whenever you want to, then you know that needs strong arms, glutes, quads, core and back.

Your daily activity plan will include, each day, some form of exercise that is specifically designed to help you increase the strength of those specific muscle groups. In this regard you are no different to an elite athlete. To get the most returns on the time and effort you invest you need to be very specific in what you want to achieve which means you need to be clear in why you want to achieve it so that it has real meaning for you.

If you do all that, all that is left then is to "go for it". Break down the exercises you need that will give you what you want and then put that plan to work every single day.

Is it really that simple? Yes and no. Yes it is because from a certain perspective you just need to choose an end goal that truly means something to you, put together the exercises you need to achieve it and yes, over time this approach will get you there.

At the same time you need to be patient, persistent and be kind to yourself. If what you want was easy to achieve you would not need any of this planning. Because it is not easy to achieve you need this structured process to get you there and along the way there will be moments when you will lose heart, you will feel you are failing you may tell yourself that the effort involved is too much and that you are swimming against the tide.

This is where you need to be kind to yourself. Understand that losing heart at some point, that getting tired of always trying is natural. We all have dark moments. We all experience dips in our mood and become momentarily disheartened. There are no exceptions to this.

Embrace those moments too. Accept they will happen and that they are a natural by-product of the process. By accepting them without blaming yourself of failing you learn to embrace your momentary weakness and use kindness to yourself to become stronger. This is the clearest signal of the internal changes you have made that make you mentally as well as physically stronger.

The old you. The one who didn't know about the three-step process and could not work out how to articulate the end goal never mind reach for it would have folded at the first sign of weakness, at the first misstep. This is not you right now though.

You know how to achieve empowerment over your life and control over your choices which means you have control over your actions. From here on you can only get better.

Take Action

Problem: Although we all know we should exercise we find it very difficult under normal circumstances to get round our natural aversion to stressors like physical exertion.

Solution: We can get round this most of the time by reframing the way we feel about exercise. The operative word here is "feel". If we're no truly feeling it we are unlikely to take action. Even if we do take action in the short term we are highly unlikely to stick to it. In order then, for us to "feel" why we are exercising we need to define its emotional value to us. What is exercise there to do, for us?

Action Plan

You may want to use pen and paper for this exercise but it can also be done, equally well maybe, in your head.

Feel what it is you get out of exercise. Not the obvious things: strength, speed, stamina, a way to control your weight. These are just by-products of physical activity. Feel what it is that exercise gives you by understanding how you feel before, during and after exercise.

Once you have it clear in your head, articulate it: Exercise is necessary for me because ..... [Fill-in your own blank]. Write it down somewhere, even on your phone. Carry it always with you as a reminder and read it to yourself in those times when it feels difficult to exercise because you're just not in the mood.

There are eight DAREBEE workouts that follow. These are workouts that have been developed to help you feel better in your body without disrupting your day, tiring you out more than you are already or requiring you to have special equipment, a lot of space or special clothes. Integrate them in your day as necessary and slowly get into the habit of using them every time you want a quick pick-me-up.

daily MOBILITY

DAREBEE WORKOUT © darebee.com
Repeat each exercise **6 times**.

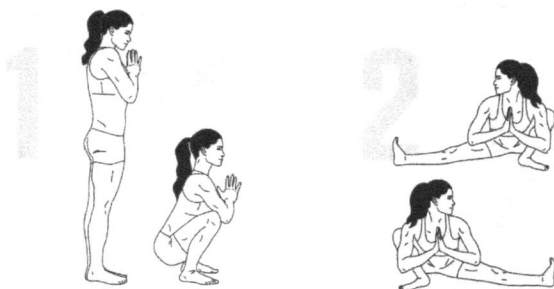

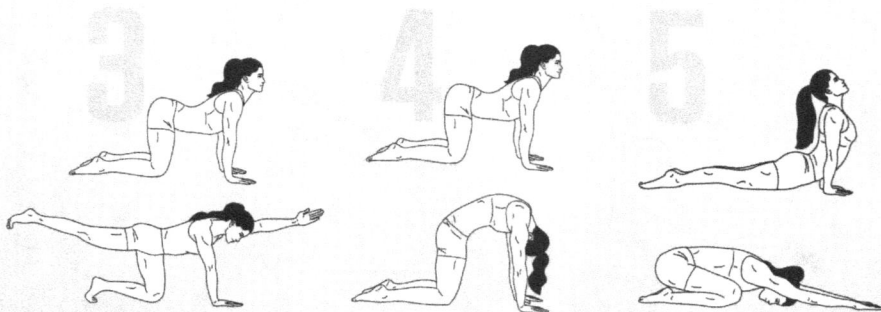

ANTI-AGING
MOBILITY

DAREBEE WORKOUT © darebee.com

LEVEL I 3 sets **LEVEL II** 4 sets **LEVEL III** 5 sets **REST** up to 2 minutes

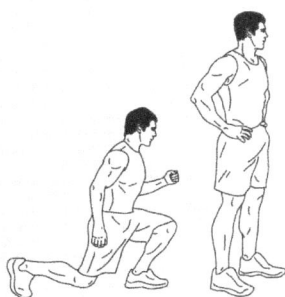

10 reverse lunges

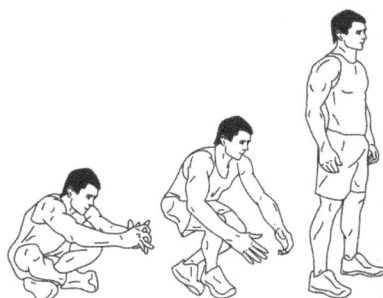

10 sit-to-stand

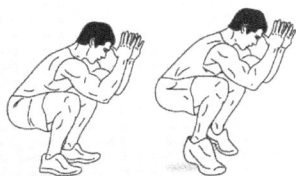

10 squat toe rolls

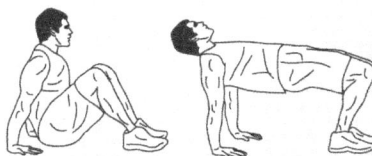

10 full bridges

NECK

DAREBEE WORKOUT
© darebee.com

IN COLLABORATION WITH **NHS** choices

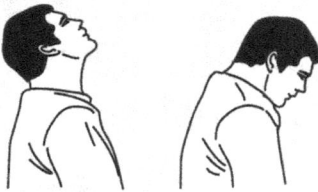

10 back and forth tilts

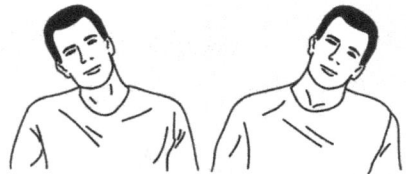

10 side-to-side tilts

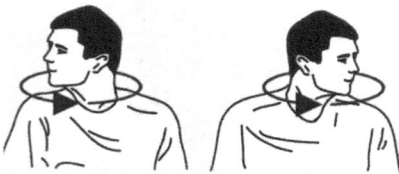

10 neck rotations

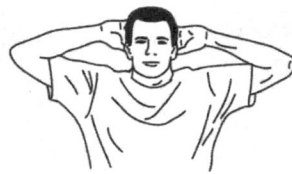

10-count press

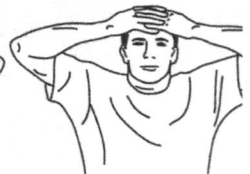

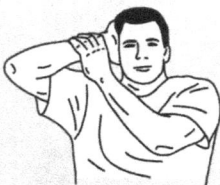

10-count press

10-count alternating side press

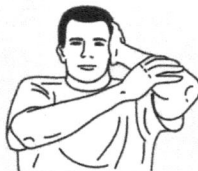

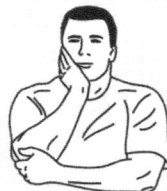

10-count alternating chin press

movie night

DAREBEE WORKOUT © darebee.com
repeat every 20 minutes during a movie

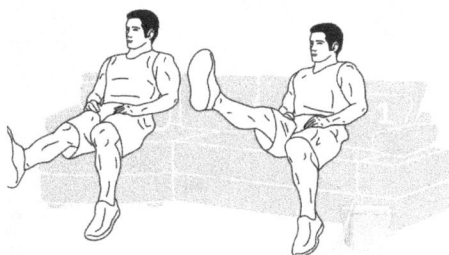

10 leg swings

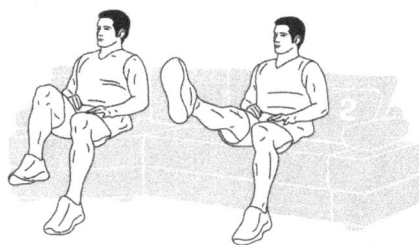

10 front snap kicks

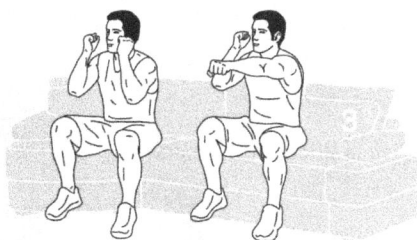

20 punches

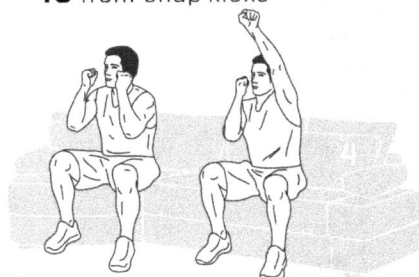

20 overhead punches

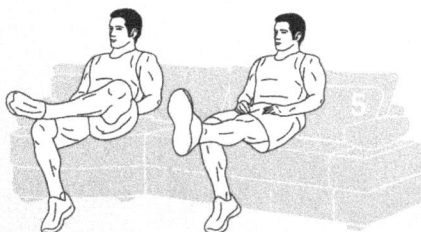

10 knee taps

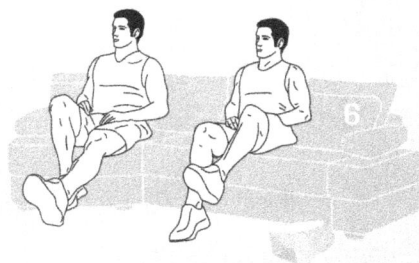

10 air bike crunches

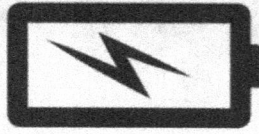

ENERGIZER

ENERGY BOOSTING © **darebee.com**

12 reps each exercise

repeat once whenever your energy levels are low

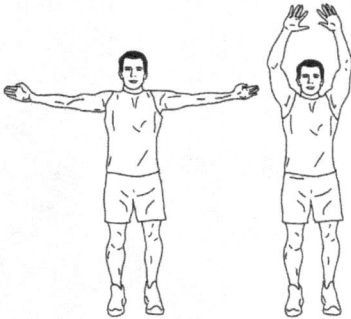

arm raises

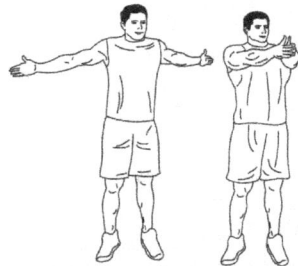

chest expansions

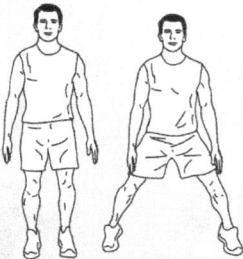

half jacks

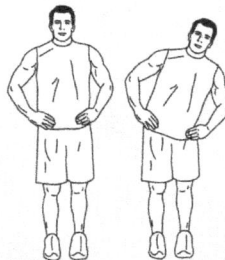

side bends

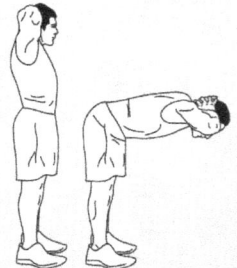

forward bends

POSTURE PERFECT

DAREBEE WORKOUT © darebee.com
repeat 3 times | up to 2 minutes rest in between

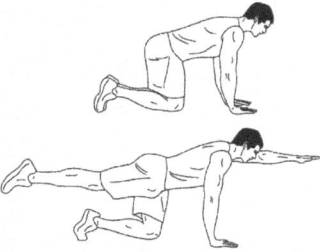

10 alt arm & leg raises

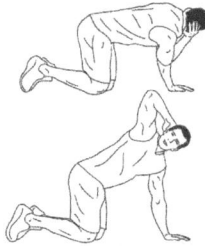

10 plank back rotations

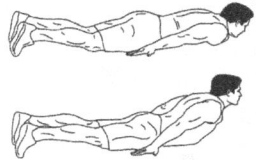

10 prone extensions

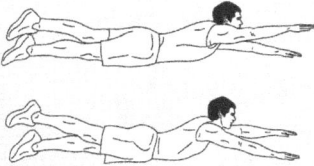

10 swimmers

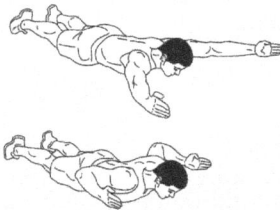

10 W-extensions

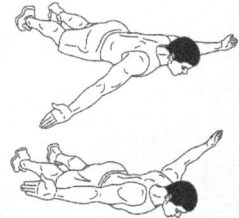

10 prone reverse fly

JOINTS
SUPPORT

DAREBEE WORKOUT © darebee.com

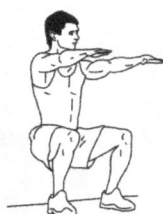

10-count wall sit

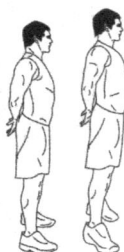

10 calf raises

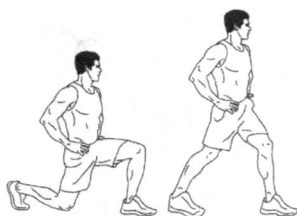

10 split lunges

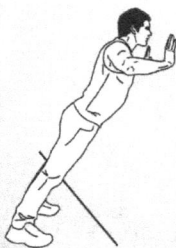

10-count wall push-up hold

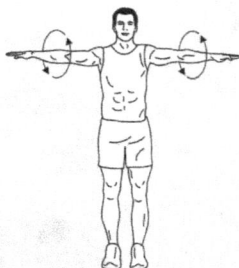

30 raised circles

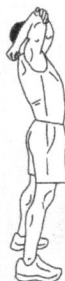

10-count shoulder stretch

breathe
easy

WORKOUT by © darebee.com

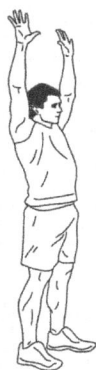

Arms above your head

1) Breathe in deep;
2) Hold to count of five;
3) Exhale to count of five.

Repeat 5 times in total.

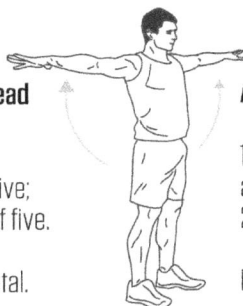

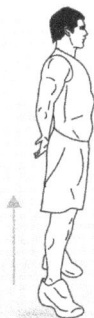

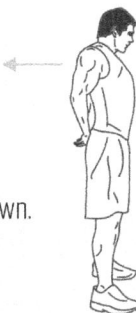

Arm Raises

1) Breathe in
as you raise your arms;
2) Exhale on the way down.

Repeat 5 times in total.

Calf Raises

1) Breathe in as you rise;
2) Hold to count of five;
3) Exhale as you drop down.

Repeat 5 times in total.

Shoulder Stretches
arms behind your back

1) Breathe in as you stretch;
2) Hold to count of five;
3) Exhale as you relax.

Repeat 5 times in total.

The following four DAREBEE workouts are short. They're perfect to use as a way to decompress after a hectic day when you don't feel like working out intensely or as workouts that are there to help you regain your inner balance. They can also be used as back-ups on days when you don't feel like exercising but still need to do something to help your body and mind feel alert.

morning
BREATH
WORK

BY DAREBEE © darebee.com

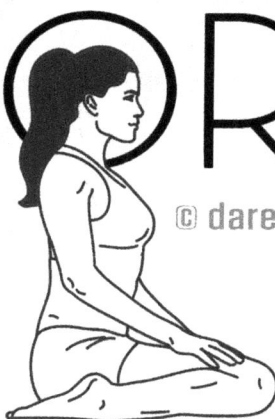

30 seconds
1-2-3-4-5 count slowly breathe in.
1-2-3-4-5 count slowly breathe out.

2 minutes
1. Inhale deeply through the nose.
2. Exhale slowly through the mouth.
3. Repeat until the times is up.

Finisher
1. Inhale deeply through the nose.
2. Exhale to 90% & hold for as long as you can.
3. Inhale fully, hold & count to 15 then slowly exhale.

FACELIFT
WORKOUT
by DAREBEE © darebee.com
Repeat each exercise 5 times.

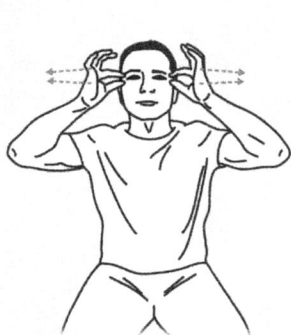

Draw parallel lines above
and below your eye with
your fingertips or nails.

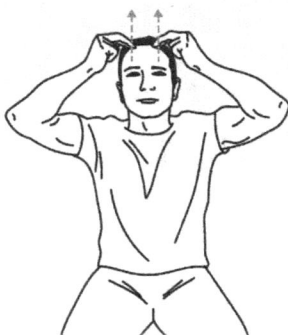

Start from your eyebrows
and stretch your forehead
towards the hairline.

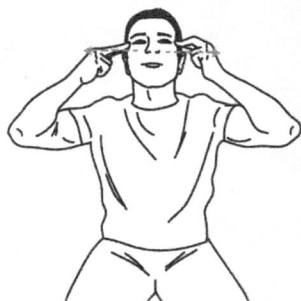

Start from the edge of your
eyes and stretch the skin
towards your hairline.

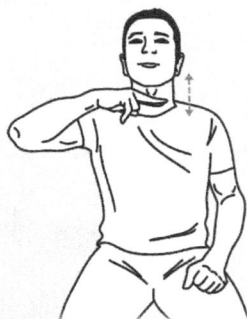

With extended index and
trigger fingers together
tap rapildy under your chin.

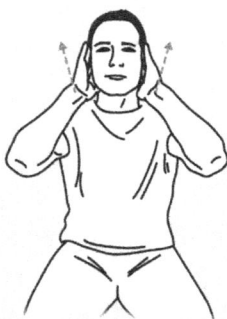

Place thumbs under your jaw
and move your hands firmly
towards the top of your head

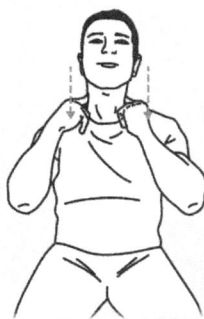

Place your index finger behind
your ear and pull firmly to
the base of your neck.

Breathing
Workout

by DAREBEE © darebee.com

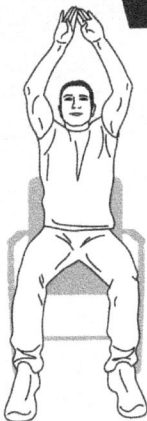

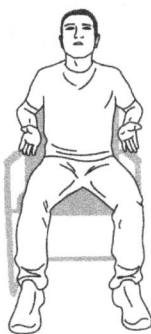

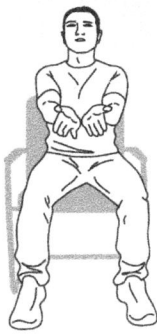

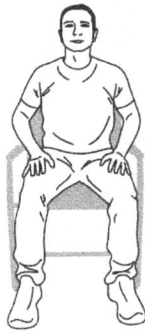

Breathe in slowly, hold to a slow count of ten then exhale slowly. Repeat 3 times.

Take ten rapid breaths. Hold without breathing to the count of twenty.

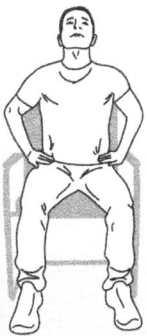

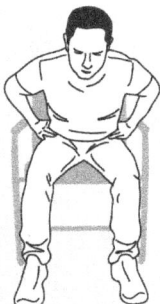

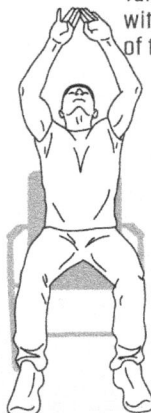

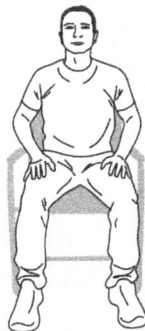

Breathe in and lean back, breathe out and lean forward. Repeat 3 times.

Breathe in fast, breathe out fast. Hold for count of three. Repeat 3 times.

PANIC ATTACK

RECOVERY

DAREBEE MINI WORKOUT © darebee.com

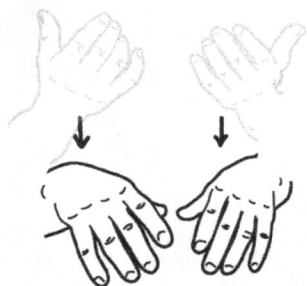

Count: 5-4-3-2-1
while shaking your hands rapidly.

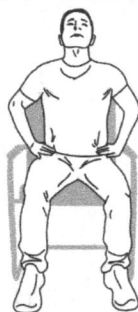

Count to 10 & hold.
Expand your chest,
shoulders back, hands on hips.

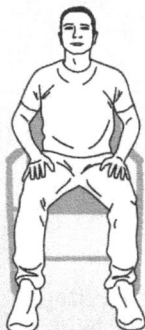

Take a very deep breath.
Take a shallow breath
immediately after.
Breathe out slowly.

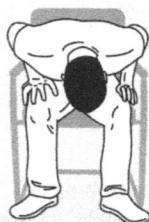

Count to 20
while holding the fold.

THE HIDDEN ORGAN

We are everything we can think of. The problem is most times we end up thinking so very little of who we are and who we want to become that we never really get the chance to think ourselves into something other than what blind chance, circumstances and our immediate environment dictate to us. This makes us feel frustrated and resentful. We project our own failings onto the world, shift the burden of responsibility beyond us and feel that someone other than ourselves somehow, owe us something.

Let's start this chapter with a question, again: How does aging manifest in the body? How do we know a person is 'old' just by looking at them? If you are like most people who answer this question you will most probably say that "hey, we know a person is old by the amount of white hair they have on their head, or their lack of hair if they are balding, by the quality of their skin and by the general shape of their body."

Indeed, visible hallmarks of aging include pigmentation problems on the skin, poor skin texture, lines and wrinkles and a certain amount of flabbiness that is the direct result of muscle loss.

Most of our immediate sense of old age has to do with appearance.

We may look at physiology. Watching someone move slowly, with a poor sense of balance who is exhibiting evidently low muscle strength can lead us to conclude that they are what we usually call "old and frail".

Again, our perception of aging in this case is based upon an externally observable physical performance.

While we readily apply these judgments on what we see with our eyes when we observe other people's physical appearance or the way they move we don't apply the same label when we look at someone who is thinking or someone who is making a decision.

We think and we make decisions with our brain. Much like hair or skin or bones or muscles or tendons or ligaments, the brain is an organ that is subject to the physical laws of degradation and aging.

More so than all the other organs I would argue because it is both more complex and it is involved in virtually everything we do which means it works all the time and usually does more than one task at a time. This makes it vulnerable to aging because small, destabilizing effects can have serious repercussions that set off a cascade of other events.

What we call 'aging', our perception of all those externally observed factors that make up the bulk of our criteria for our decision to call someone "old" is the manifestation of a number of hidden factors that gerontologists and biologists call the true hallmarks of aging.

The twelve most agreed upon hallmarks of aging are: genomic instability, telomere attrition, epigenetic alterations, loss of proteostasis, disabled macroautophagy, deregulated nutrient-sensing, mitochondrial dysfunction, cellular senescence, stem cell exhaustion, altered intercellular communication, chronic inflammation, and dysbiosis.

Each of these, as you might guess, unfurls into a complex field of scientific research on aging that studies how cell function and cell structure changes over time inside our body. We are able to better understand some of the underlying mechanisms involved in aging because of our ability to observe their external manifestation: the loss of youthful traits like thick luxurious hair and soft skin. The loss or impairment of physical attributes like strength and balance and mobility. The loss or impairment of some of our basic functions like vision, hearing and taste.

Yet, despite the apparent complexities involved in the study of the intracellular and cellular mechanisms involved in all this, we still mostly fail to consider the impact of all these changes on the human brain.

Much as it remains the center of the awareness of our existence and the anchor point of our perception of the world the brain inside our head manages to stay out of sight and considered only when things go so drastically wrong that we have observable, physical manifestations of its malfunction. By then, of course, it is usually too late to do much about it.

We will do better than that here. Instead of waiting to experience the aging of the brain through a reduction in the quality of thinking which often leads to a reduction in the quality of life, we shall, in this chapter, look at what we can do to help our brain stay as young and healthy as our body.

To do that successfully we must first look at how the brain gets old and what this aging means from a practical perspective. Only then can we really understand what interventions are available to us that will disrupt the brain's aging process and how we can apply them.

Brain Power

Most of us who drive have, at some point in our life, driven down a two-way, two lane road with cars parked on the side we are driving on and traffic coming at us the other way. And we have all, in that context, slowed down a little bit but squeezed through the narrow space available to us without scraping up against the cars parked on the side of the road we are driving on and without having a head-on collision with traffic coming the other way.

None of us in that context, I hope, have felt the need to stop the car and leap out in traffic to measure the width of our car and then measure the width of the space we have to squeeze through in order to drive down that road. But if we didn't do that how did we know that it was OK to squeeze through? How were we able to calculate the space and position of our car in such a way that it would go through the gap available to us, with sufficient clearance on either side so as not to cause a head-on collision or damage other people's parked cars?

If you drive I know I have you thinking about a skill that all drivers take for granted. But even if you don't drive here's another example for you to think about that makes use of a similar situation. Without the use of a mirror brush your teeth. Using a toothbrush to brush our teeth is an activity we all habitually engage in at least twice a day.

We do so without having to see where our teeth are located, where the toothbrush is in relation to our face and the position of our mouth and without having to visually check how wide our mouth is when open. We can do it without the use of a mirror, in the dark or even while we are actively engaged in other tasks such as reaching for a hand towel, walking around the house or one-handedly scrolling through our phone.

We manage to engage in all this amazing multi-tasking dexterity with barely any conscious effort on our part because a complex number of processes take place in our subconscious brain which model our body, the tools we use on a regular basis and the three dimensional world we live and work in so that they can all seamlessly come together.

Inevitably, and a little bit reluctantly on my part we need to get a little more technical at this point to better understand how all this actually happens, but I will try and keep things as simple as possible and provide clear, plain language explanations whenever complex technical terms come up.

Beyond Our Grasp But Not Beyond Our Reach

If you've ever played billiards or pool you know immediately what I am talking about here: you hold some kind of foreign object in your hand, in our example a pool cue, but in other contexts it could be a long stick, a mechanical extender of some kind or some other kind of grappling or prodding tool. You're now tasked with affecting another object which you want to grab or move which is beyond your grasp, but not beyond your reach. You do that through the transmission of mechanical energy from your body to the object you want to affect via the object you hold.

Seeing how it's taken a paragraph just to describe something so simple you understand there is a deep, underlying complexity guiding all this. The laws of physics are at work conserving energy and momentum, transferring motion and changing the direction of mass. To describe all this correctly it would require exact measurements made by precise instruments, complex mathematical calculations describing the laws of mechanical motion originally formalized by Isaac Newton and a clear understanding of geometry and gravity.

Yet, we do all this with barely a thought. The rawest pool player begins, after a game or two, to better understand angles and momentum, transfer of energy, acceleration of mass and gravity. All this is done through feelings: sensations that are picked up and transmitted by the body's network of nerves to the brain that processes them into a signal that tells us what's going on around us.

How all this magic happens is no less than miraculous and it is important to understand it if we want to have a long, healthy and happy life.

Predominantly there are three key processes that are at work:

- Representation
- Distal Attribution
- Embodiment

Collectively they are incorporated into a Schema. Schema is the term given to any cognitive framework or concept that describes a pattern. A pattern, in this case, is a model of connections with a certain repetitive structure to them that renders them instantly recognizable. Think of it like a knitting template you use to create a quilt by blindly following the repetitive structure of a few design elements.

Schemas are a representation of the underlying actualities we use to interpret the world. The brain too employs a Schema to make sense of the

80

virtually infinite variety of sensations it experiences through the reporting of the vast network of nerves that runs through our body. Neurologists and neuroscientists call this, appropriately, Body Schema.

The Body Schema allows our body to use our brain to map where it is at and how it feels in relation to the external world. We employ Schemas because they are a shortcut. Instead of trying, each time to make sense of each one of the complex variety of signals that we receive from the vast network of nerves from our body our brain uses the Schema it has already stored to make sense of the world quickly.

When we sit down on a hard bench it is the Body Schema effect that interprets electrochemical signals send by our nerves which then tell us that the bench is cold, hard on our butt and therefore uncomfortable. When we bend down to tie our shoe laces it is Body Schema that informs us just how far we need to bend down and how far to extend our arms in order for our fingers to complete the dexterous task.

Body Schema is active in everything the body does and to do its work it employs a sixth sense that tells it exactly where the body and its boundaries are. This sense is called proprioception. Proprioception is like magic. Without our being aware of it at all it tells the brain exactly where each part of the body is, even when we cannot see it.

To give you an example, try putting a chain around your neck with one of those clasps that require you to pull back on a kind of small lever for the clasp to open and a loop to be fed in. It's called a lobster claw clasp because it kind of resembles a lobster claw.

Guaranteed, the first time you try with your hands behind your neck, you will fail. You can't see what you're doing so you're trying to guess the positioning of the clasp and the loop. Your fingers will cramp from trying to keep the lobster claw open long enough for you to thread the loop holding the other half of the chain through. Your neck, shoulders and upper arms will ache from the effort as you hold your arms in this unnatural position. It takes a lot of concentration to do all this. You will feel sweat break out in your brow. You may want to take several breaks and upwards of ten minutes to do it the first time.

But the time after that it feels easier and you do it a little bit faster. The time after that it is faster still and way easier. Five days in of doing that and you can do it with virtually no thought, while walking around your home and talking to a friend on the phone.

This is a perfect example of proprioception at work. Your brain processes signals you are unaware of; that tell it the exact angle of your elbow and shoulder joints and the exact positioning of your wrists required to bring the two halves of the lobster claw successfully together.

Body Schema uses proprioception to then safely navigate the external world, which in our example was your home, without bumping into any of its walls or furniture. If you ever watched the 1999 breakout film *The Matrix* there is a scene, early on, where the protagonist, Neo, attempts to navigate a crowd crossing the road at pedestrian lights in what they call "a training program" and he bumps almost into every person in his way. That's because he doesn't yet have good proprioception between his digital, projected, self and the real him and his Body Schema is still poorly developed.

By the time we're all old enough to go out in the world on our own we are all capable of successfully making our way through a crowded pavement without bumping into anybody. We make this happen through Body Schema that employs one or more of three processes available to it. In no particular order these are:

Representation. As the name suggests Representation implies a kind of internal modeling of the external world. Imagine, for a moment that the body is a machine and you are its pilot. You are encased at the topmost part of it, in a totally dark cell. The only way you have of controlling this machine then is to look not outside through a couple of tiny slits you have but inside where a three-dimensional model of the body is formed and then, around it, there is an ever changing three-dimensional model of the world. It is only by looking at this ever-changing picture that you, the pilot, can make decisions whether the machine you control will lift its arm or its leg or will bend down or reach up and how high or how far each move must happen.

This is a gross oversimplification of a very complex process but it gives you a good idea of how Representation works and what it does.

Distal Attribution. This is the second process at work and it allows the body to experience something that happens at a distance, even if it's through a foreign object like it is happening to the body directly.

Gamers are intimately familiar with it. Play a first person shooter on Playstation and while you're using your fingers to press control buttons and your thumbs to guide mini joysticks, your brain is engaged in controlling hands and legs on the screen running around a digital environment, handling weapons and squeezing triggers. It doesn't end there. Fishermen waiting for fish to nibble at the bait on the end of their hook, feel every tag and nudge like it's happening to their hands and not experienced at the point of the fishing line, attached to the fishing rod they're holding.

This is a much similar sensation to that experienced by blind people who report that the sensations of the tip of their cane as it explores the area around them feel, to them, like they are part of their own body.

Distal Attribution has, two more parts to it each of which makes perfect sense the moment we examine it: Peripersonal Space and Extrapersonal Space. Peripersonal space is the area immediately around our body and how we perceive it. Extrapersonal Space is the area beyond our physical reach and how we perceive it.

Gamers, again, watching themselves climb a steep hillside on screen feel part of the effort required and their physical responses match that of their on-screen avatar even though they are sitting in their home rather than climbing a mountain.

They may not be physically out of breath and their muscles may not get tired but such is the power of the mind to mirror a perceived external reality and bring into it the brain's modeling capability that their body's biochemical responses are very similar to them doing the real thing. If you're a fan of *The Matrix* you already know that moment when Neo, having failed his first test inside the matrix and fallen from his jump realizes that what hurts his digital self also hurts his physical self: "Your mind makes it real". If you haven't seen it, suffice to say that there is a sizeable body of research that shows that sitting still and visualizing a specific exercise in detail leads to neuromuscular changes that reflect what happens to the body when we actually perform that exercise. Distal Attribution is all of that.

The third and final process via which the brain incorporates something that is not of itself into its Body Schema is called Embodiment. Anyone watching a Samurai wield a Katana, or a virtuoso violinist play their instrument with their eyes shut feels that they are watching someone using an instrument with the same degree of dexterity and control that we have over parts of our own body.

Embodiment was believed to be a process during which the brain incorporates an instrument or a tool into the Body Schema like it is an organic part of itself. The latest research has shown that this is not the case. The brain is all too aware that the instrument or the tool an expert is using is not part of their body but it develops neural pathways that allow the person to manipulate that instrument or tool with the same degree of dexterity and control as it actually is part of their body.

I must stress that Embodiment requires a high degree of familiarization and control that comes only with many hours of concentration and practice.

This concludes, for now, the technically difficult parts of this section of this book. It was necessary to examine these because they show, most clearly, that when it comes to physical movement, including exercise, the brain plays an incredibly important role in the body even though it is the body's involvement we are aware of and not the brain's.

We see that when circumstances dictate it the brain changes first and then the body follows. The changes that take place because of exercise are of two types: Neurogenesis - when the brain forms new neurons and neuroplasticity when the brain changes the way it is wired and structured so that it can behave differently.

If the brain can change because we exercise our body and make it stronger, in a similar pattern when we age and become weaker it is the brain that is affected first and then the body even though, again, it is the body that carries the visible signs of aging.

We cannot thrive, at any age, if our brain is not in peak condition or if, at the very least, it does not have the four key requirements for good brain health. These are: sleep, nutrition, exercise and social activity.

The first three of these are identical to what is required for a healthy body which only serves to highlight how linked body and brain really are.

This book is about practical interventions we can apply in order to age on our terms as we get older so that we have improved quality of life in our later years and to do that we need to feel both empowered and in control. None of this is possible without taking the necessary action to protect, nurture and develop our brain so it can continue to function, at peak capacity, as we age.

The final section of this chapter is all about that.

Protecting The Brain

What's the first image that comes into your mind when you think of soldiers in a war zone? Or ancient Greek warriors on a battlefield. Or American Gridiron Football players? Or workers on a construction site? Beyond the uniforms and the equipment what is common in all these images is the use of helmets.

We understand that in any theater of human activity that has the potential of creating unexpected situations and hard impacts, we can damage our brain and we therefore try to protect it.

The use of helmets drives the message home: what we do here is potentially dangerous. We need to exercise special care.

Yet, no special care is taken when it comes to the brain in relation to what we eat or drink or how often we exercise or how well we sleep. Because there are no moving parts to the brain we often don't realize when it gets tired and needs a break and we always fail to understand what can distract it, what can exhaust it and what can harm it.

Walk down a dark alley in a part of town you don't know well, alone, in the middle of the night. What do you feel? If you are an average human being you will feel a sense of anxiety and even fear. The fact that it is dark and isolated will make you feel physically vulnerable. Your heart rate will go up. Cortisol levels in your body will rise. Your heart and lungs will work harder pushing more oxygen and blood into your muscles. Your surface body temperature will rise as a result. You may feel some sweat in the palms of your hands. Your stomach may tighten. All your senses will go on alert. At a neurochemical level, whether you consciously know it or not, you have been activated.

All of this will happen before you detect a threat for which you will need to take action. If there is no threat evident and you do not have to take action then what are you reacting to? The answer is that all of the things you have experienced, physically and emotionally as you go down that dark alley are the response to the perception of your brain.

Faced with a novel situation with a high uncertainty factor and a lack of real world information the brain goes on high alert and takes the body with it so it can be prepared to face a potential threat.

When something that is only an unrealized possibility can affect us so much, imagine what happens to our brain when we eat something like junk food that is certifiably bad for it, and our body.

We all love junk food. We all love it because it has three ingredients our body is programmed to seek: fat, sugar, and salt. Here, again, we encounter ancient responses and drives that are meant to help us if we lived in an ancient world but which today cause us only harm.

In our distant past our hunter-gatherer ancestors encountered a meal that contained high amounts of fat or sugar or salt as an occasional event brought about by hunting skills and chance. Food was perishable. Lacking refrigeration and sophisticated preservatives the best way to capture the nutrients it provided to us was to consume it.

The human body has an infinite capacity to store fat for a reason: it's the best way to store and transport fuel for the times we will need it. In the modern world of course we can pop into a supermarket and come out in minutes carrying enough calories to support a group of those hunter gatherers of our ancient past for a week.

The moment we eat junk food or food that is low in fiber and is, therefore, easy to digest and high in fat or salt or sugar, we directly cause changes in the gut's massive population of bacteria. The changes in our gut population of bacteria, in turn, affect the hormones they produce, impact directly on the neurotransmitters that activate our central nervous system and increase gut inflammation.

We will talk about inflammation, its root causes, and effects and when it is good or bad, at length, in the next chapter. Here, it is enough to say that inflammation in the gut is not a good thing. It is a precursor to a host of other systemic problems that destroy our health and the fact that we cause it by eating the wrong things shows just how much we still need to learn, as a society, about practices that help us remain strong and healthy throughout our life.

A single meal of junk food certainly affects us but it is consistency that does the real damage. Consistently bad food choices and poor eating habits lead to persistent inflammation in the gut. There are only two organs in the body that have their own independent nervous system, an indicator of their importance not just to our physical but also to our neurological and therefore mental health. The heart is one. The other one is the gut. The task of the gut appears simple: coordinate absorption of nutrients from the food we eat and then enable motility and secretion. But the neurons of the gut independent as they may be of the central nervous system are not isolated. They are in frequent communication with the brain.

It is this channel of communication that creates the pathways through which what we eat influences how we feel and, eventually, how we think. And because the brain is so involved in how we move, everything that affects it then also affects our fitness and, as a direct result of that, how we age.

The chatter between the gut and the brain, we now know, is multi-faceted. In the most obvious way it takes place via the vagus nerve that runs from the brain to the gut and reports to the former the state of play of the latter. But it also takes place through the release of hormones, neurotransmitters, metabolites and immune cells. When so many different elements are required to work in relative harmony for the smooth operation of two important organs like the gut and the brain we realize that the connection is delicate and relatively easy to disrupt.

Inflammation in the gut, unchecked, impairs its function and provides that disruption. The effects this disruption can have can vary and though subtle to spot at first they are both wide ranging and pretty devastating: There can be a reduction or complete stop in the brain's capacity to create new neurons, what we call neurogenesis. The brain's ability to reorganize its neurons in new patterns and learn new skills, for instance, can also be impaired or be completely stopped. At a cellular level the tiny engines in our cells called mitochondria that are responsible for the oxidative phosphorylation process that generates all the adenosine triphosphate (ATP) we use as energy can also be compromised making us feel listless and dispirited. The body's immune system may be compromised making it harder for us to shake off viruses like the common cold and making us more susceptible to more serious infections. There is even evidence that mood swings, depression and even leaky-gut syndrome which is linked to a host of neurodegenerative conditions are directly linked to a disrupted gut/brain axis and changes in the gut's bacterial populations as a result.

Clearly there is a lot at stake. More than we would at first think.

None of us want to age as we get older. Also none of us want to feel that we can no longer rely on our brain to remember things, understand things, make good decisions and help us make choices that lead to good things for us.

Alarming as all this may be, at the same time, it is really encouraging. It shows that if we want to enjoy long-term fitness and health if we want to truly build ourselves to last we can start with the brain before we even get to the body.

We can employ strategies that safeguard our health and allow us to feel that we can control our body and that we can control our life through our decision-making, without making a large investment in time and money.

What are these strategies? What actions should we be taking? Some of these will sound familiar because they are the exact same ones we use to keep our body fit and healthy:

- Sleep
- Exercise
- Nutrition

But the brain is the body's most complex organ. It has additional requirements so to these three we shall now add a fourth:

- Social Activity

Each of these activities will look different for each of you. How well you put them to use will depend on the demands made on your time and energy by your lifestyle, your job, your age, your sex and even by where you live.

If you want to be healthy and feel strong and live a long life however there is a baseline you need to aim for.

To create that baseline, we will start with the what, the actions you must take for each of these requirements and we will see the 'why' as we go along. This way you can most easily customize everything to what you can do to help your brain stay young, healthy and strong and by association give your body the best chance possible to remain strong, feel healthy and age slower.

Step One To Great Brain Health: Sleep

When we sleep the brain repairs itself from the damage caused by stress, bad food and alcohol. It uses the hours of the night when we are not awake to strengthen the connections it needs for better physical responses when we are awake and to forge new connections so we can remember the thing we learned, both physically and mentally. This is what we call neuroplasticity.

That new Tik-Tok dance you learned? It only becomes real for you after you sleep and your brain remembers the dance routine and can reproduce it any time, anywhere. The new cooking recipe you memorized? Or the chapter of the How-To book you read? Again, without sleep you will not remember them.

Sleep is important for improving memory. It is also important for improving behavior. When we've slept enough we have better self-control. We are less impulsive in our decisions and less likely to lose our temper and overreact.

Impulsive decisions and over-reactions contribute to our feeling captive to circumstances and events. Feeling captive to circumstances and events increases the sense of anxiety we feel and the amount of toxicity our internal organs are exposed to. This downward spiral is broken by simply getting more sleep. And making sure we sleep well while we do sleep.

To sleep well you need three basic ingredients:

- A good sleep schedule that prepares you to wind down for the day.
- Avoid stimulants like caffeine or depressants like alcohol for up to eight hours before bed time.
- Avoid reading the news or following social media, activities that excite specific areas of the brain, before bed time.

Poor quality of sleep and not enough sleep are linked to inflammation in the brain, poor energy management in the body (which over time can lead to obesity and diabetes), heart issues and dementia. Poor quality sleep inhibits neuroregeneration and repair.

Step Two To Great Brain Health: Exercise

Exercise is turning out to be preventative medicine. It helps prevent our body and brain from breaking down and sickening and it helps improve what's broken and sick. All forms of exercise help us maintain our body younger and stronger and a younger, stronger body helps our brain remain sharper.

We don't have infinite time to exercise so if we have to make a choice for our brain health some forms of exercise deliver better results than others.

These are:

- Walking
- Dancing and martial arts
- Meditation and Breathing

Ideally you want to do all of them. Walk as often as you can for as long as you can. Do some form of dancing even if you can't dance and just hop around to music at home or some form of martial arts and, meditate and engage in breathing exercises.

If you are not sure how to meditate the QR code on this page will give you an easy guide anyone can follow. If you have never done breathing exercises before there is also a QR code for a breathing workout that will immediately revitalize how you feel.

QR Code for better breathing

QR Code for meditation

Step Three To Great Brain Health: Nutrition

You don't need to have a personal nutritionist nor do you have to be a food scientist yourself to know what foods help your brain health and what to avoid to help your brain work better.

To help you improve and maintain great brain health the foods you eat should do the following:

- Fuel your brain.
- Help it reduce inflammation.
- Help it fight high blood pressure.
- Help it protect the integrity of its neural network.

If you cut out sugary foods and sugary drinks, including soft drinks, you are on the right track. If you reduce fatty foods and alcohol you're also giving your brain a better chance to stay healthy.

None of these steps that protect your brain health are difficult but because all these foods are easily available and socially acceptable it requires a lot of intentional thinking and some planning so that we can resist their allure when we find ourselves in a social situation where they are plentifully available.

We need to be able to diplomatically turn them down without appearing to cast judgment on those who consume them and without turning this into a rejection of people some of whom we will obviously care about.

Finally when it comes to knowing what foods and drinks to include consider: nuts and seeds, avocados, tomatoes, blueberries, ginseng tea, green tea, coffee, tumeric tea and berry juices.

The list is not exhaustive and, at the back of this book, in the appendix section there is a more comprehensive list of foods and drinks you can consume that are protective of brain health and even have neurogenerative or neuroprotective properties, in other words they either help the brain generate more neurons or protect the ones it has from sustaining damage from stress.

Step Four To Great Brain Health: Social Activity

Every time I mention this step in conversation I get the same reaction: nods, smiles and anticipatory grins. The need to be social is hardwired in us but it comes at considerable energetic cost to the brain. This is why spending time with people is often tiring and occasionally draining. It really takes a lot of energy to do.

The reason I get nods, agreements and smiles is because most people who hear the words "social activity" envision a party. So let's clarify this: being a party animal is not the same as being social or engaging in social activity.

Social activity is about engaging in two-way communication. It requires listening, understanding before talking, so every social engagement in order to benefit our brain health requires us to:

- Listen
- Comprehend
- Respond

It sounds simple when I present it like this but listening to another person talk and truly understand not just what they are saying but why they are saying it activates the parts of our brain that recall memories and knowledge of the real world which are then used to interpret the context of our social engagement in the present.

We call this ability "social cognition" and it's the total of mental skills we use to make inferences of what is going on inside other people so we can understand their feelings, thoughts and intentions.

You know that 'gut feeling' you have had about a person where without any evidence you can point to at all you feel like you shouldn't trust them? That comes from all those hidden psychological processes that make up social cognition.

The point is that there is a lot of psychological activity and mental processes that are happening in a social context and they require energy in order to happen. It's like a workout for the brain and, like any physical workout, it is tiring. It triggers adaptations we don't see but whose effects we certainly feel and, over time, it makes socializing better but not easier.

The best way to see social activity or socializing is as a team sport. You just cannot successfully do it on your own. Like any team sport it takes us out of our comfort zone a little and forces us to learn to trust other people. Just like any team sport socializing delivers better results the moment we surround ourselves with high quality people.

The friendliest game of basketball you can imagine can turn pretty hostile and pretty stressful, very quickly if you have people on the team who are toxic, have big egos and want to win at all costs. Apply the same issues across a dinner table or a gathering of people at a party and the results will be just as hostile and just as toxic and just as stressful as in the basketball game of our example.

So, when it comes to socializing make the same choices you would if you went into a team sport to play a friendly game for fun:

- Be there to have fun and enjoy the experience
- Pay attention to everyone there not just yourself
- Choose people who are agreeable to hang out with

Just like with team sports do this often and it will feel better and you will get better at it. Just like with team sports there is never an ideal day and time to socialize or an ideal group of people to do it with. It is important that you do it regularly and find for yourself the small group of people who are your tribe. The people who 'get you' and who in a pinch would have your back and be able to give you the moral and psychological support you need.

What's important to remember is that socializing is an important element of your fitness routine designed to keep you healthy and happy for as long as you live. With this in mind we are ready now to examine if there is such a thing as a "fitness recipe" you can apply in your life, no matter what stage you're at.

Take Action

Problem: Whenever we think of fitness we tend to think of the body and only of the body and we completely neglect the brain. Yet mental health is central to our physical health.

Solution: The brain and the body are an indivisible whole. When our body is physically tired our brain underperforms. In everything we do by way of fitness and exercise we must now factor in the brain and its requirements: the fuel it needs, the rest it requires and the socializing that is necessary to help keep it healthy. All of these have to be planned activities so that there is a consistency to them.

Action Plan

Use a calendar to plan your week and then plan your month. Input the days when you will exercise and the time you will spend exercising. Add days when you will socialize. In each set targets: what do you expect to get from your exercise? What are your goals in each social outing?

Plan your month like a project whose outcome is to produce a mentally healthy and physically capable human being at the end of it.

Do not be overly ambitious in your aims but be consistent in your actions. Once you have the habit of planning your week and your month you will notice that you now also have a greater sense of control over your life.

There are eight main DAREBEE workouts that follow, as always, after a chapter. These workouts are specifically designed to help you develop stronger neuron signalling pathways and improve the body/brain connection. Again, there is a customizable element to them which allows you to adapt them to your fitness level and needs. Most are without equipment. As always, pay attention to the illustrations on each workout and the rest time you are given.

CIRI

DAREBEE WORKOUT © darebee.com

LEVEL I 3 sets **LEVEL II** 5 sets **LEVEL III** 7 sets **REST** up to 2 minutes

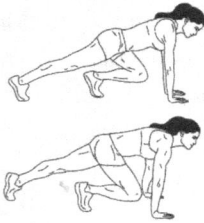

10 climbers

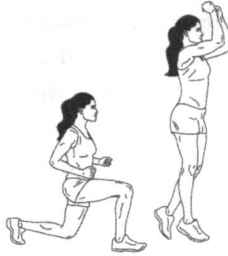

2 jumping lunges

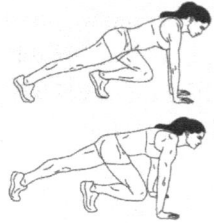

10 climbers

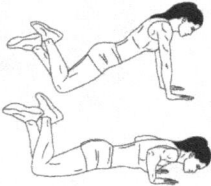

2 knee push-ups

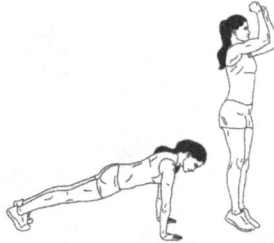

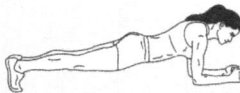

10 basic burpees

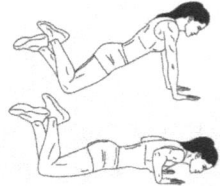

2 knee push-ups

10-count elbow plank hold

GREYWALKER

DAREBEE WORKOUT © darebee.com

LEVEL I 3 sets **LEVEL II** 5 sets **LEVEL III** 7 sets **REST** up to 2 minutes

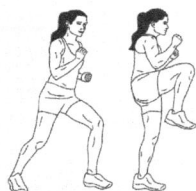

20 knee strikes

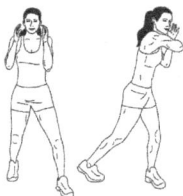

20 elbow strikes

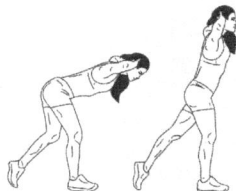

10 staggered deadlifts

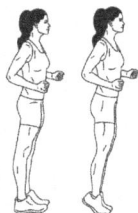

20 calf raises

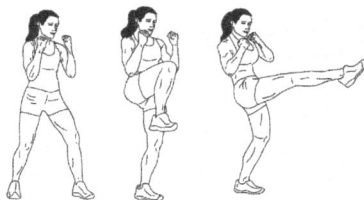

20 front kicks

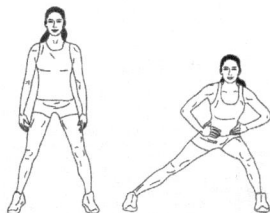

10 side lunges

HEPHAESTUS

DAREBEE WORKOUT © darebee.com
2 minutes rest between exercises

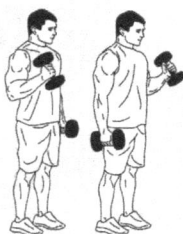

12 hammer curls
x 5 sets in total
20 seconds rest
between sets

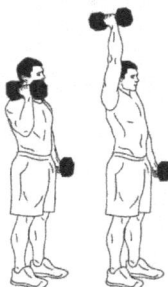

12 shoulder press
x 5 sets in total
20 seconds rest
between sets

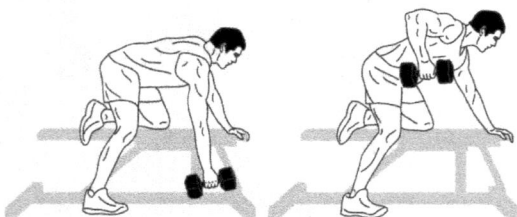

12 rows
x 5 sets in total
20 seconds rest
between sets

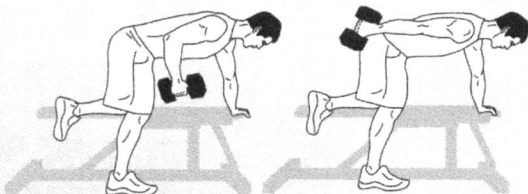

12 tricep extensions
x 5 sets in total
20 seconds rest
between sets

500 KICKS

DAREBEE WORKOUT © darebee.com

turning & side kicks | 500 kicks in total
split into manageable sets

SIDE KICKS

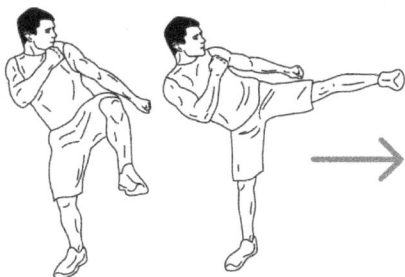

TURNINGE KICKS

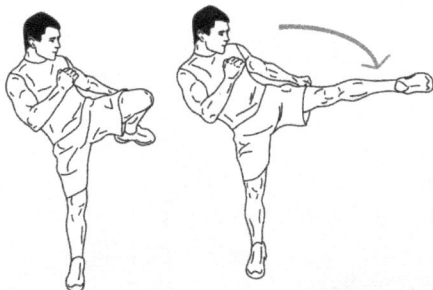

LIGHTS OUT

DAREBEE WORKOUT © darebee.com

LEVEL I 3 sets **LEVEL II** 5 sets **LEVEL III** 7 sets **REST** up to 2 minutes

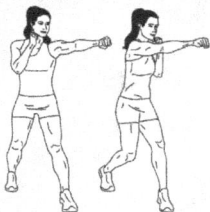

10 punches

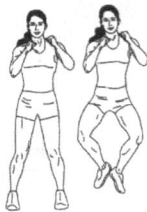

3 hop heel clicks

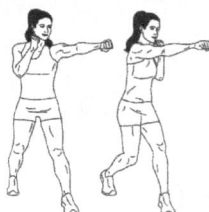

10 punches

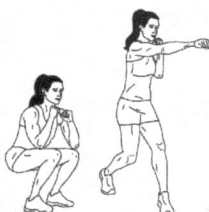

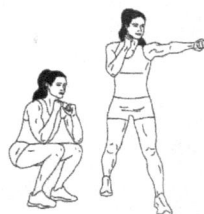

10 squat + punch

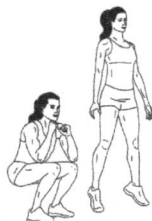

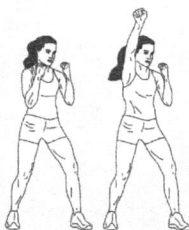

3 jump squats

10 squat + punch

10 overhead punches

SUPER HIIT

DAREBEE WORKOUT © darebee.com

Level I 3 sets **Level II** 5 sets **Level III** 7 sets | 2 minutes rest

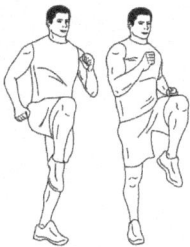

20sec high knees

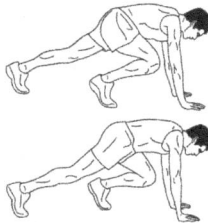

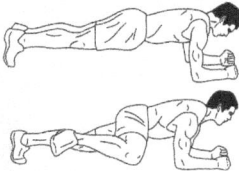

20sec climbers

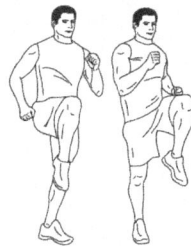

20sec high knees

20sec plank crunches

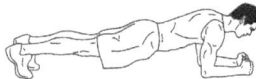

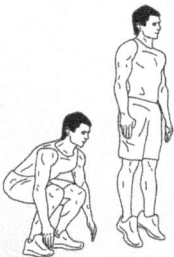

20sec plank hold

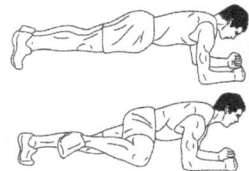

20sec plank crunches

20sec jump squats

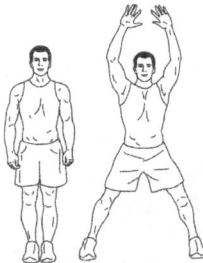

20sec jumping jacks

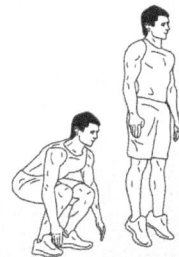

20sec jump squats

INDOOR
CARDIO

DAREBEE WORKOUT © **darebee.com**
repeat 5 times   up to 2 minutes rest between sets

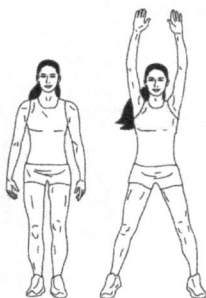

20 jumping jacks

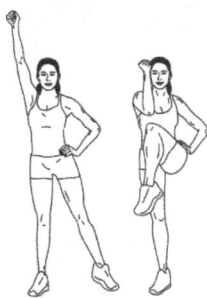

10 knee-to-elbow

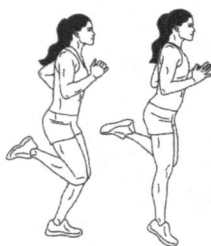

10 butt kicks

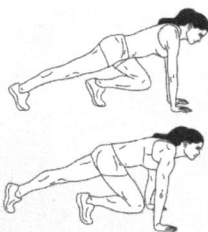

10 climbers

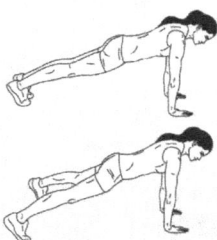

5 plank jacks

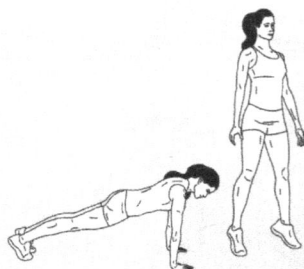

5 basic burpees

Cardio High

DAREBEE WORKOUT © darebee.com

LEVEL I 3 sets **LEVEL II** 5 sets **LEVEL III** 7 sets **REST** up to 2 minutes

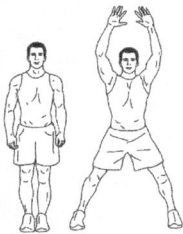

20 jumping jacks

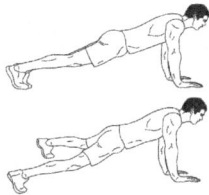

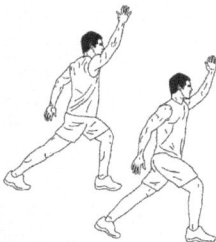

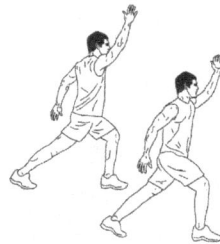

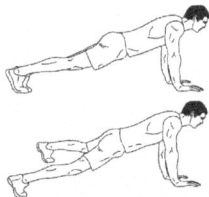

20 plank jacks

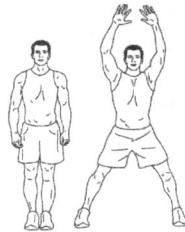

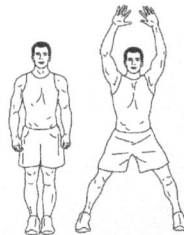

20 jumping jacks

20 split jacks

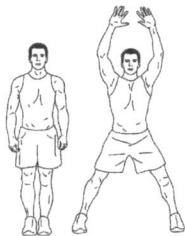

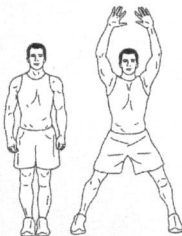

20 jumping jacks

20 split jacks

20 jumping jacks

20 plank jacks

20 jumping jacks

There are, again, four customary DAREBEE workouts that follow that are of lighter intensity and also make less of a demand on your time. The four workouts chosen here have been field-tested as all DAREBEE workouts and focus on mental strength, inner balance and well-being. They can be used instead of a main workout when you are low on time and energy or they can be incorporated in your daily fitness and well-being practice.

BRAIN BOOST

WORKOUT by DAREBEE © darebee.com

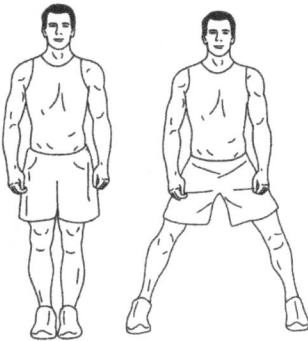

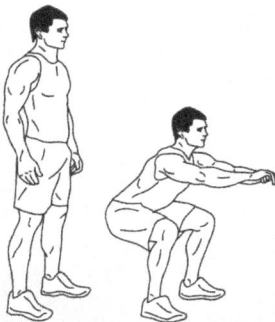

10 half jacks

2 squats

10 half jacks

2 squats

10 half jacks

2 squats

10 half jacks

2 squats

10 half jacks

2 squats

done

binary
workout
by DAREBEE © darebee.com

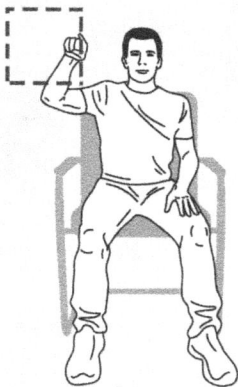

Draw a square with the extended finger of one hand.

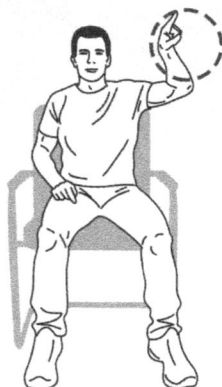

Now draw a circle with the other.

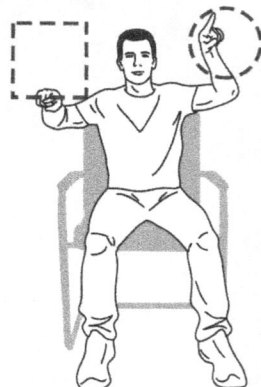

Now do both.

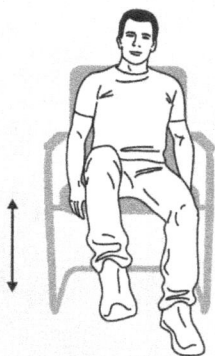

Sitting down raise dominant knee up & down.

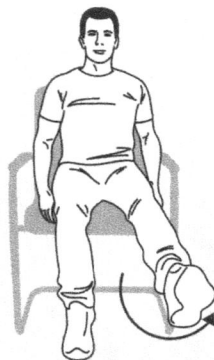

Kick the other leg back & forth.

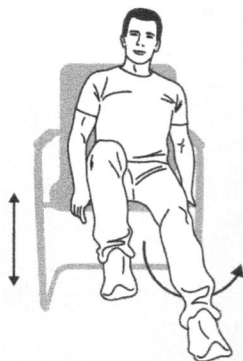

Now do both.

WILD FIVE

DAREBEE CARDIO WORKOUT
© darebee.com
LEVEL I 3 sets
LEVEL II 4 sets
LEVEL III 5 sets
2 minutes rest between sets

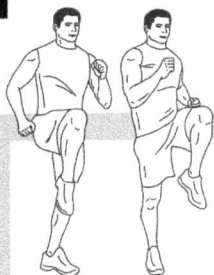

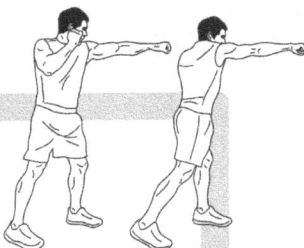

REST

1 minute high knees
1 minute punches
1 minute high knees
1 minute sit-ups
1 minute high knees

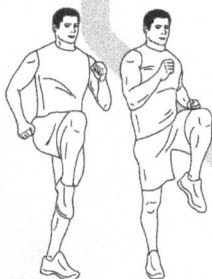

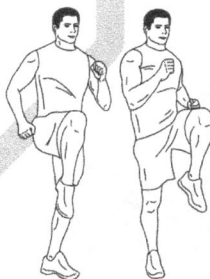

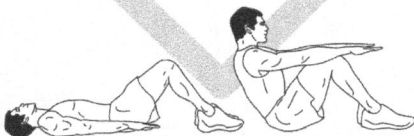

balance yoga

DAREBEE WORKOUT © darebee.com
Hold each pose for 30 seconds then move on to the next one.
Repeat the sequence again on the other side.

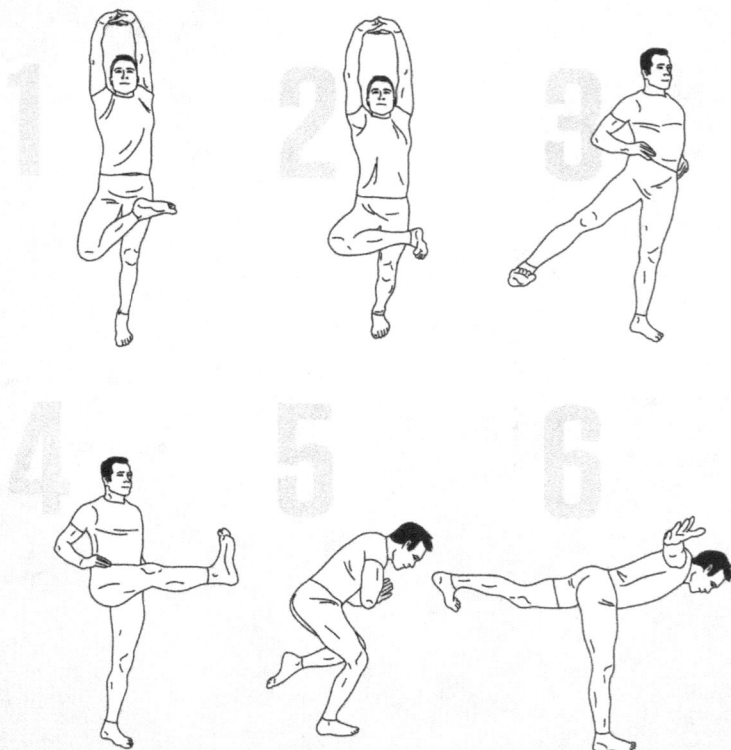

THE FITNESS RECIPE

You can never understand what you cannot record. You can never improve what you cannot measure. And you can never control what you cannot analyze.

Can there be such a thing as a fitness recipe? I mean can there be truly a series of actions we can undertake and a series of choices we can make that will help us get fitter no matter what? And, if there is such a thing already why isn't everyone one doing it? Why is everyone still struggling with their fitness?

If I answer these questions backwards you will see immediately why 'the secret' of a fitness recipe is not really a secret at all. We have always known what to do but we have not always felt we can do it. Sometimes we allow ourselves to believe the excuses we are so adept at creating. At other times we simply don't want to face the added responsibility of taking charge of our own physical fate and our own physical health. We may not feel capable enough, or smart enough or knowledgeable enough or committed enough or disciplined enough.

Whatever the excuse strategy we use the end result is usually the same: we end up not doing what we should be doing because we have managed to find a "good enough" excuse that gives us the permission we seek to not do what we know we should do.

To top it off, because deep down we know we are just using excuses every time we don't exercise enough, don't eat the right things, don't sleep right and don't socialize, we feel uncomfortable about our choices. So, we end up feeling guilty about it all. And because we feel guilty and guilt is a core emotion that governs social behavior we end up getting caught in yet another downward spiral where we try to avoid the very same things that can helps us stay young and active.

The Challenge Response is what happens to the brain and body when we are faced with a physical (or mental) challenge. When we experience guilt the Challenge Response kicks in. Our blood vessels dilate (vasodilation), sending more oxygenated blood to our brain and muscles. The adrenal gland releases a shot of cortisol which increases the amount of stress we feel. All of this, left unchecked builds up. Our blood pressure goes up. Insulin levels that regulate the amount of sugar in our bloodstream are reduced. The way our body processes food and stores it into fat goes in overdrive.

Guilt, which is a negative emotion that is designed to help us moderate our social responses and regulate them in coordination with others is also associated with the neurotransmitter oxytocin which, in a communal; tribal setting, leads us to enlist the help of others.

Unfortunately when we experience guilt inside our self for our own failing and we have no support network to help us we are alone. We feel all the bad emotion associated with it without having any option to relieve them through communal sharing or by talking it out with people we can trust.

So what happens next? Obviously, because we feel bad because we are failing to exercise regularly, eat food that is good for us, sleep right and socialize enough, we go even further out of our way to avoid even acknowledging that these problems exist.

How many times have you heard the phrase "Sleep when you're dead" as a way of exonerating and even rewarding with some kind of imaginary social badge of honor, those who fail to look after themselves adequately and sleep enough? Or "This is my Cheat Day" when it comes to diet, usually said by someone who's about to gorge on ice-cream and chocolate, sugar-laden foods that will physically stress the body's insulin response and will do very little by way of nutrients?

"Cheat Day"? What does that even mean? The person who says that is only cheating themselves. So how is that OK to use as an excuse?

To avoid all this, ideally, the perfect fitness recipe would have us feeling good all the time about our self and it would make it as easy as possible for us to do what is right for us in terms of exercise, sleep, nutrition and the all-important socializing.

To make it even more perfect it would be the perfect recipe to apply to anyone no matter their age, sex, experience or level of fitness. In other words it has to be a one-size-fits-all recipe that truly fits all and is easy to keep.

Well, that recipe has two main ingredients and some extra spices that deliver a number of benefits which we shall examine in this chapter. But the primary ingredients are called "Sustaining" and "Sustainable" and in this section we shall explore the first one.

If what you do to make yourself feel strong and be healthy is not good for you both in the short term and long term, doing it makes zero sense.

I don't care if you run marathons and clock up a sizeable number of miles each week. If that is not good for your physical, mental and psychological help if it is not helping you wake up full of zest for life and full of energy to face the day then what you are doing has no real future.

It is that simple.

You will ask, and quite rightly, what should I doing? What is it I must be doing if I have no idea what to do in the first instance?

To work out what you should do consider the three primary, basic things we need to be physically healthy:

- Strength
- Mobility
- Aerobic capacity

And the three things, again, that combine to give us the physical, mental and psychological changes we need:

- Exercise
- Nutrition
- Sleep

You can be any one: young, old, man, woman, rich poor and any combination in between. It doesn't matter who you are, it doesn't matter how fit you are, it doesn't matter if you have not yet started your fitness journey.

What matters is your ability to bring together the elements that will sustain you in your life journey. Are you strong enough to do the things you want to do in your everyday life without injuring yourself and without exhausting your muscles? Are you mobile enough to get around your day, to bend down and pick something off the floor and get back up quickly again? Are you able to grab a bag of groceries and walk a mile with it to get it to your home?

If you can do all that, you then have a great basis to build on for a long and healthy life. If, however you struggle, and that is most people today, take heart from the fact that there is still time for you to fix this.

The human body is amazingly responsive to external stimuli. We are unique amongst all the animals on the planet in our ability to change both inside and out to function better in the environment we live in. The ability to adapt is one of our superpowers.

This means that with a little planning and persistence you can change what you can do and you will then also change how you feel. To trigger the adaptations you want so that you feel in control of your body and able to do all the things you want, you need to incorporate a little more physical activity in your everyday life.

I am not talking here just about exercise. In the course of your daily life you must plan some non-exercise related, physical activity. Here's the thing about fitness: there is no autopilot fitness program that can be implemented blindly to get you to your destination. To get the most out of what you do you need to be aware of it and do it consciously, mindfully even. Provided you do it this way, if you exercise, studies show you will get up to twenty per cent more from the exercises you do in terms of adaptations that improve your physical fitness than if you did not pay much mind to what you did.

Even more crazy is what happens when it comes to how you think about all the other stuff you do in your day, each day of your life. If you have the mental attitude that sees all the things you do in your life as a positive experience that helps you become stronger and better and that includes all your day-to-day physical activity, then your body helps you become fitter and stronger. The opposite is true if you do not have this positive, mental attitude.

In a defining study on hotel maids carried out by the Department of Psychology at Harvard University, the researchers showed that when the hotel maids were separated in two groups and one group was told that their everyday work activity, the cleaning, bending and lifting they were engaged in, counted as exercise and helped them get fitter they showed a decrease in weight, blood pressure, body fat, waist-to-hip ratio, and body mass index while their colleagues who were performing exactly the same tasks but had not been told that these tasks contributed to their fitness, showed no physical change at all.

That was a study on hotel maids. If you are a little bit dismissive, and you shouldn't be, of that sample of the general population, for whatever reason, there is a further study carried out by the Department of Psychology at Stanford University, this time alongside the Warfighter Performance department at the Naval Health Research Center in San Diego on aspiring Navy SEAL recruits undergoing the grueling Basic Underwater Demolition/SEALs training that's seven weeks long.

The fourth week of that seven week-long training course is so physically, emotionally and psychologically demanding that it is more popularly known as "Hell Week". SEAL recruits are already "the best of the best". By the time they get to the beginning of their course they've been weeded out so the ones who undertake that course are physically fit to a very high standard and mentally focused. Yet, the attrition rate of Hell Week is a staggering 75%.

Three quarters of all those who try to become Navy SEALs do not get through that fourth week despite outwardly, at least, all of them being fairly close in terms of physical capability. The researchers wanted to understand the difference.

What they saw was that the ones who actually made it through saw everything they did in a different light to those who dropped out. Successful recruits saw the physical difficulty of the trials they had to get through as making them stronger physically, mentally and psychologically despite the fact that the activities had been designed specifically to break the recruits down, physically exhaust them and demoralize them.

The ones who failed, who dropped out saw the activities they were engaged in as something that ground them down and weakened them in body and mind.

The physical fitness of the recruits who dropped out and the ones who succeeded and passed was very similar. Just like with the study that recruited hotel maids, the ones who succeeded however felt that the activities they were engaged in were helping them become better and they were fully invested in them.

In this most convincing two examples of the power of mind over matter, the studies suggest that how you feel about what you do transforms the effect it has on you. That's what exercise being sustaining also means. Do you go to the gym? If you see it as drudgery, if all you can focus on is how tired you are from your day to day life and how much more tired this makes you and how hard it is when you get there, then it is not sustaining. The chances are that you will be one of the people who add to the statistics that show how many people stop exercising after a few weeks and then either don't exercise again or exercise too little to do them any good.

Sustaining then is the label you use to hang everything under, that makes you feel good even if what you do is physically difficult and makes you feel momentarily stressed or tired. Everything we can place under this label can just as easily be placed outside it: long walks, hard exercise, ice baths, sauna, running in the heat or running in snow, taking a flight of steps, walking to the grocery store, playing with your kids.

It is within your grasp to magically switch what each of these activities and pretty much every activity you can conceive of that you engage in, does for you. All you have to do is change how you feel about it.

'All' I say, but I know it's not a small thing. To change how you feel about what you do you have to understand how you feel about yourself. You have to use optimism and a positive mindset to flip what you experience so that the stressor of the moment does not change the potential benefits you can receive from the stress that you experience.

This is how you engage in sustaining physical activity.

What you do is up to you. How it affects you however depends on how you see it and if you see it in the right light then its positive effects are undeniable. Just as it is undeniable that anything that is sustaining is also sustainable.

Sustainable

Imagine breaking rocks for fun. No matter how you cut it, it is hard physical work which traditionally, within the penal system was designed to systematically grind you down physically and mentally as part of your punishment by society. If you engage in it as a hobby, outdoors and I don't know of anyone who does, I'm willing to bet any money that it's not the kind of hobby you engage in for life no matter how strong it may help you get. It's simply not designed to make you feel good.

Similarly, your fitness journey, the things you do that will help you remain physically strong, mobile and aerobically fit for as long as possible, have to be lifelong activities which make you feel good when you engage in them and are capable of being adapted to your needs as those needs evolve and change.

We already know that physical exercise is a stressor. Exercise needs to be physically hard enough for us to feel it as a stressor so it can trigger the physical adaptations we need to become fitter and remain fitter. We already know we are hardwired to avoid stressors, so there is a real need to logically reconcile these two drives in our minds now.

If our only way forward is to seek out and engage with stressors that we have been biologically programmed to avoid it seems like we are forever locked into an internal fight with ourselves. On the one hand we want to exercise and be physically active all the time because that will help us feel strong and be healthy. On the other, we seek to avoid all of that.

Let's examine the "sustainable" strategy a little closer to see how we can square this circle.

When we were kids we never did anything that didn't feel good to us. Child behavior is predicated upon doing and feeling and observing and copying which then leads to doing and feeling in order to test the behavior that has been observed and copied.

It's a simple method that, over time, leads to more complex behavior patterns but it is based upon the basic sense of what something feels like. Actions that don't lead to good feelings are quickly abandoned and actions that do are reinforced and refined.

This is a gross oversimplification of course but it serves us well here. Children are directed in their learning by their environment, their feelings and, obviously, the adults who are responsible for them.

Back to us now.

Adults are a little more complex. Our own learning strategies include a memory of our childhood where we learn through a stimulus/reward pathway. But to that we also add two additional layers of complexity. One is external and it's called Connectionism and the other is internal and it's called Cognitive Field.

As the name implies Connectionism reinforces or inhibits learning in adults based upon our understanding of our standing in relation to others around us and society at large.

Cognitive Field, on the other hand, suggests that we learn because we can reorganize some of our understanding of the world around us and achieve a better sense of mental clarity.

What does any of this have to do with exercise, good health and longevity? Plenty. Just like we are unlikely to truly engage in any kind of long-term activity that is not really good for us (i.e. one that is sustaining) we are also unlikely to engage in any kind of long-term activity that is not easy to implement (i.e. it is sustainable from an effort required point of view).

The complex ways through which adults learn are necessary because the world we inhabit is also complex. Navigating it on a daily basis is tiring. Dealing with its everyday issues and the occasional crisis that happens is exhausting.

And now, on top of all this, we have to exercise.

Exercise, by nature is an energetic activity. Whatever we do is going to use up energy and we have only a limited amount of energy available to us each day. This leads us to the first deep truth about exercise: In the modern world exercise is an energy management system we implement for the body and mind. Nothing more.

Will it help you lose weight? Directly, no it won't.

Is it really designed to make you stronger or faster? Again, not really. These are the things that happen as a result of exercise and it is easy to say that correlation is causation because exercise is the only tool available to us that will bring about these changes but these changes are the result of a deeper, underlying reality. That reality is how the body uses, stores and manages energy.

The body is designed to survive. Without the body there is no brain. Without the body/brain union there is no us. Everything the brain does is about survival. Everything the body does is about survival too.

The brain and the body have different mechanisms they put in operation to help us survive. The one thing in common all these mechanisms have is the same thing that has been behind every successful evolutionary adaptation we have gone through. Take your pick: opposable digits, bi-pedalism, speech, a larger brain, a body that has no naturally strong muscles, binocular vision, REM Sleep there is more on this list, but you get the picture. All of these adaptations that create a unique organism we identify as human; decrease, by a tiny amount, the energy required to perform a specific task.

Collectively all these changes represent a significant amount of energy savings. All these changes are, therefore, efficiencies that are created in order to give the body and brain the best possible chance of survival in a world where energy is always an issue.

I know we don't live in that world any more. You know it too. But our body and brain are ancient. Even those of us born yesterday have been built following a genetic blueprint that kicked into operation some 300,000 years ago when Woolly Mammoths and Saber-toothed tigers still roamed the Earth.

That genetic blueprint still operates like there are no supermarkets filled to the rafters with calories waiting for us to just enter and consume them, no cars to help us get about and no building that can protect us from the heat and the cold. Instead, that genetic blueprint, expects us to face periods of food scarcity and a daily exposure to predators which we must either hunt down or run from.

Here's how that blueprint which has been designed through evolution to give us the best possible chance of survival trips us up today: Take two groups of people who are given two different types of backpacks to carry. To remove any bias, both groups of people are told the same thing about the backpacks: that they contain equipment that monitor walking gait.

One type of backpack weighs about 20% of the bodyweight of the person carrying it. The other type of backpack is filled with foam and is considerably lighter. Each group is then asked to estimate the distance to a particular point in the horizon.

This is called visual perception and because of our ancient hunter/gatherer past we are quite adept at estimating distance under normal circumstances. The introduction of the weighted backpacks in the mix however adds an additional physical stressor, so the situation for some of those being asked to estimate the distance is not exactly normal.

When this field experiment was carried out, everyone in the group with the weighted backpacks overestimated the distance to the landmark and overestimated the effort required and time it would take for them to walk there.

This is the ancient energy-saving protocol that run us at work, tricking us into overestimating the difficulty of something so we become less likely to engage in it, when we are tired.

Apply this now to a situation you face: the prospect of having to get a workout in at the end of a busy day, or the idea that you will have to go to a social gathering after a full week of hard work, or the thought that you need to just drop down and do ten push-ups at the end of the day before you go to bed. The chances are that you feel rising inside you a resistance that is hard to articulate in words but which is that all-familiar feeling that translates in your brain as: "This is hard", "I don't feel like it", "I'm too tired to do this today".

All the excuses, in other words, that we use to not exercise when we should. All the excuses we use to not socialize when we should. All the things we tell ourselves that let us off the hook because we strongly want to be left off the hook because of this wave of resistance we feel rising up inside us.

Since this resistance to exercise, especially when we are tired is natural it would appear that our efforts are doomed. No matter what we plan to do when we are rested and our batteries have been fully recharged, we are bound to fail the moment we get caught up in the complexity of our life. There appears to be no hope.

Fortunately this isn't so for two reasons: first, because in this particular case the ancient mechanism of our body has provided an additional means for us to overcome this handicap of its ancient logic and second, because we are smart. We have the capability to rewire ourselves through the employment of knowledge and clever strategies.

First, however, some good news from the world of neurobiological research. Researchers at the Spanish Cancer National Research Center (CNIO) discovered two specific proteins that are expressed by muscles when they start to work. These proteins activate the muscle/brain pathway and make us want to keep on moving our body once we start to move it in the first instance.

There is ancient logic in this too. In the distant past of our ancestry when all these pathways, drives and imperatives were formed by evolution and engraved in our biology, those of us who survived were the ones who managed to keep our body moving in order to escape danger or successfully hunt, even though physical activity was energetically expensive and a stressor we wanted to avoid.

What it means for us today is that no matter how bad we think we feel and no matter how tired we think we are, the moment we start to exercise changes take place in our bloodstream and proteins are expressed by the muscles themselves that activate the parts of our brain that keep us doing more of what we are doing already.

It would appear that the trick then is to "show up". Turn up with the intention to do what we can for however long we can. What will always happen next is that we find that we can always exercise more than we think we can and we enjoy it more than we think we will.

The first rule for this to happen is: Show Up!

The second rule is: Make it Easy.

Because we are hardwired to feel averse to physical activity when we are tired or think we have a lot to do we need to plan our physical activities in a way that makes them accessible no matter what.

There are countless examples of how we complicate our lives. I will give you two that most people use: the first one is The Obstacle Course.

The Obstacle Course kicks in when we provide a solution to our need to exercise but then proceed to put up any number of barriers to it.

Suppose, that we choose to join a gym. This will naturally require paying a gym membership fee. That's one obstacle. But now we also need to travel to it and how we get there is an obstacle in itself: do we need to walk? Can we drive there? Is there traffic to negotiate when we do? Can we get parking? What's the weather like? Will it be busy when we go?

Already the obstacles pile up just on that and we haven't even got started yet. Then there is the attire we need: special shoes? Weightlifting gloves? Headphones for our music? Special gym clothes? Towel?

More obstacles.

On a day when everything has gone our way and we feel good about ourselves we throw everything in a gym bag, leap in the car and go and train. But on a dark winter evening with the rain pelting outside and the indoor heating set to a super-comfortable setting, going out to exercise seems like a massive venture in itself. It only takes one setback in our personal life or a manic day at work to derail our fitness plans because "we are too tired", "it's too cold", "we are exhausted" and we shall "make up for it next time".

What if, for those days when these things happen at work or the outside elements are against you, you had a contingency plan ready? Things you can do at home to keep you on track and help you maintain your fitness regardless? Exercises that require no equipment and hardly any space which you can do in your underwear if you want to?

Would that not then solve the problem for you?

Making exercise sustainable then is not about exercising on easy forever. Nor is it never getting out of your comfort zone. But it is about making sure that you are always able to exercise somehow no matter what.

For that to happen you need to have plans already in place so you know what you need to do the moment you can't go to the gym. Spending time trying to decide what to do as an alternative to our regular exercise stuff, is tiring in itself. It only helps magnify the perceived difficulty of exercising. But if you have everything in place already because you already planned for this day coming, you will find yourself automatically reaching for your contingency plan because you understand you need to exercise to remain healthy and feel strong.

Your sustainable exercise plan then is: Show Up - Get started and do something no matter how little it may be.

Have back-up plans so you can exercise even if you can't go to the gym, can't get to your dance class or your spinning class and have no equipment and hardly any space, at home.

Sustainable is just the second ingredient of our magical Fitness Recipe. How you put it together is up to you. There are brief exercises called exercise snacks at the end of this chapter, to help you. There are also workouts you can pick so you don't have to worry about what to do. Most require no equipment and hardly any space.

The second excuse most people use is The Scarcity Trap. They get fixated on what they haven't got, instead of what they have thinking, wrongly, that if they had it; it would change everything.

Here's what often comes up in this case: "time", "equipment", "a gym near me", "clothes", "spare cash", "a training buddy". The variations are endless. The theme however is always the same: I haven't got X so I cannot do Y. X can be anything you haven't got and Y, in this case, is exercise.

Again, sustainable solutions focus on the outcome you want and the resources you do have. If you haven't got time can you find five minutes each day before hitting the shower? If you haven't got any spare cash can you exercise without a gym membership, equipment and fancy clothes?

Sustainable solutions never strain our resources, either in materials or time or emotion. They're sustainable because we have used our brain to find a smart workaround the problem that we face. For that to happen of course we really need to want the outcome: we must want to exercise because we truly feel that it will help us.

We have now just two more ingredients we need to address for that perfect Fitness Recipe that will make you feel strong and be healthy all your life. The next two sections cover them both.

Inflammation Reduction

How much energy is there in your body? Science says a body at rest emits as much power per hour as a 100w light bulb. We double or triple that wattage when we exercise. To generate all this energy we need to absorb energy from somewhere.

Although we don't often think about it this way, we are true children of the stars. We feed on the massive amounts of solar power that the sun produces in its fiery furnace every single day. Because we can't absorb it through our skin like a solar cell, we ingest it instead in the form of sugars (carbohydrates), fats (fatty acids) and proteins (amino acids) which are the products of plants and animals that are part of a chain of processes that convert energy from the sun into energy we can consume and then use.

Why is all this important to us now? Because each day our body has a finite amount of energy it can safely use up. On average around 2,000 calories. In food science a calorie is the amount of energy required to raise the temperature of one liter of water by one degree Celsius. We have all that energy to use each day in order to do three things:

- Build our body.
- Repair our cells.
- Power our actions.

Cell repair and cell-building are activities that are indispensable to our long-term survival. The amount of energy used to power our actions (and that includes exercise) is also key to our health. Because all three things are important the body prioritizes energy expenditure the way a good housekeeper would prioritize a limited household budget: It looks to see what requires urgent attention and gives energy to it first.

If we were crazy enough to run 25km - 30km each day without increasing our energy intake our body would prioritize that, because obviously we need energy to move, and it would neglect essential repair and building until we started to physically break down with injuries and illness. Those familiar with intensive training routines understand exactly how this feels because they banter around terms like "training plateau" - when no matter how hard we exercise there seems to be no improvement, the self-explanatory "burn out" and "repetitive strain injuries" caused by, no surprise, repetitive strain on one body part that is experienced without adequate time or energy given to recovery and cell repair.

When it comes to spending energy for cell repair and damage repair. Some of that damage is entirely natural. If we lived in a glass jar protected from the environment with cotton wool all around us we would still experience the natural degradation of cells that need to be repaired every single day.

In addition to that we have environmental factors: radiation from the sun that affects our skin, particulates in the air that affect our lungs and germs that enter our body through cuts in the skin and through our nose and throat as we breathe.

All of these cause an inflammatory response in the body. Let's be clear: without inflammation we would die. The body's inflammatory response helps us adapt to environmental threats and fight pathogens, repair cell damage in addition it triggers muscular adaptations that we see as an increase in muscle size and strength.

Beyond the natural inflammation that cannot be avoided and beyond the inflammation triggered by the body's adaptive response to exercise there is also inflammation that is caused by lifestyle factors: alcohol, smoking, ingestion of foods rich in fat or high in gluten, poor sleep and repeated exposure to stress.

These are factors that increase inflammation in the body and brain and lead to a reduction in available energy we can use in other activities.

Modern medicine views inflammation in the body as a means of regulating the body's energy needs and considers pathologies such as some forms of cancer and autoimmune disease as the result of imbalances in the body's natural, inflammation response.

In clinical trials the energy regulation of conditions as diverse as obesity, aging and cancer is driven almost exclusively by the inflammatory response of the body's cells. In each of these the inflammation experienced by the cells plays a vastly different role and delivers a vastly different outcome.

In obesity, for instance, the body experiences chronic inflammation due to an energy surplus derived from its supply of food. This energy surplus then leads to an increase of fat-storage tissue (called adipose tissue) which also leads to fat-storage tissue hypoxia as there is a deficit between the amount of fat-storage tissue that is generated and the amount of capillaries the body is building to supply that tissue with enough oxygen and nutrients.

During physical exercise the body produces specific signaling proteins, called cytokines, that activate the process of breaking down fat (called lipolysis) to re-supply the blood and muscles with the glucose necessary to maintain adenosine triphosphate (ATP) levels in the cells so they can function.

In cases of cancer, the body experiences a high level of chronic inflammation as the immune system fights the cancer cells and the energy expenditure of this internal struggle contributes to the weight loss commonly associated with cancer.

The point is that there is inflammation taking place in the body all the time. Excessive inflammation limits the body's ability to properly manage the energy it has and reduces the overall amount of energy available to it so we become weaker.

This is supported further by a study carried out by researchers at the Neuroimmunology Laboratory, Symptom Research Department of the University of Texas. The researchers looked specifically at reduced energy availability and reported feelings of chronic fatigue by people suffering from persistent, low-grade inflammation.

Their conclusions were that persistent low-grade inflammation led to poor functionality in the body's cells, gross inefficiencies in function and an overall increase of the body's energy expenditure of as much as ten per cent.

This, in turn, made it difficult for the body to find sufficient energy for physical activity and even daily tasks, leading to reported symptoms of chronic fatigue and an inability to budget energy for exercise and the development needs of a healthy body.

By avoiding excessive inflammation we give our body the best chance possible to regulate the energy that is available to it each day and we make it easier on ourselves to use that energy for purposes that benefit us, like maintaining our health and improving our fitness.

Bear in mind that low-grade, chronic inflammation plays a key role in the development of noncommunicable diseases that threaten our survival. Cancer, cardiovascular diseases and neurocognitive degeneration that leads to developing Alzheimer's and dementia are often the result of lifestyle choices that cause low-grade chronic inflammation.

None of this is of any real value to us if we cannot now answer the simple question: How do we reduce excess inflammation in the body?

There are three practical ways:

- Exercise
- Stress Reduction
- Anti-inflammatory diet

What type of exercise? Walking, Stretching and Yoga, Resistance Training using bodyweight. Before I explain why you should engage in these physical activities in particular as opposed to others (and let's be clear here: all exercise is good and even a little of the worst kind of exercise you could possibly do is better than none) it's necessary to explain how exercise makes us healthy.

Let's play a mental game. Suppose you live a perfect life, with little uncontrolled stress and the perfect diet in a perfect environment. The air is clean, the background radiation is just right, there are zero germs and bacteria to attack your system and even the sun dims down the moment you get your necessary dose of rays for your skin to manufacture all the vitamin D you need.

Would you get fat or ill in that environment? The answer is probably yes but not as easily and not as often and it would be a harder thing to do. Why? Because in that environment your body would make great use of all the energy it gets and your cells would function just as intended. You would experience little or no inflammation and you would be able to get through your day without feeling exhausted.

This is not what happens in the real world. Why? Because we eat the wrong kind of foods, sleep less than we should, drink and smoke, fail to exercise and live in a world full of germs and bacteria.

Our body is under constant attack. Our system is constantly fighting off invaders. The cells that make us who we are, are so vast in numbers and so complex in their function that they require massive amounts of energy to work properly. Part of their defense is a chemical called interferon that creates an inflammatory response that targets internal problems and external invaders.

The complexity and vastness of the system we habitually call our body, which has over 30 trillion cells, means that it overcompensates in its defense response and causes greater inflammation than it should. The logic of that is sound. It is better to fight off an invading virus or other type of germ by overreacting than not react enough and allow it to gain a foothold in our body and make us seriously ill.

Here's where exercise comes in. Exercise creates localized damage in the muscles that are being exercised which also creates inflammation in those muscles. The inflammatory response that takes place because of exercise produces a specific type of complex protein called T-cells which, in turn, reduce inflammation in the muscle.

Experimenting at this level on humans is unethical because of the potential of causing harm to a living person, so we often use mice because of the similarities of their system to ours. Research on mice has shown that T-cells help the body's immune system regulate itself. They dampen down runaway inflammation, improve the metabolic response of mitochondria, the tiny engines inside each cell that help power it, and also shield the muscles from the inflammatory effects of interferon.

T-cells do this as a result of the cumulative effects of exercise. So no single bout of exercise, for instance, is going to bring about any improvement. But consistent periods of exercise change the way the body's immune system responds in the body and change the way cells allocate and use energy.

Both of these actions help our body remain true to its function and avoid hiccups. Which brings us to a small truth: all exercise is good for us.

When it comes to reducing inflammation in the body however some exercise is better than others. Why? Because exercise itself causes inflammation and the more inflammation is caused by exercise the more the body has to struggle in the initial phase, to deal with it.

Exercise that produces less inflammation is therefore better to implement when the goal is to reduce the overall levels of inflammation in the body.

Walking is a low impact aerobic exercise that helps the body reduce its excess weight over time and improve its metabolic efficiency. Yoga and stretching, are also low-impact types of exercise. They improve mobility and trigger muscle adaptations because of mechanical tension.

Bodyweight resistance training helps develop strength without the introduction of a constant, non-negotiable external stressor such as an added weight in the form of dumbbells or barbells. Bodyweight exercises spread the load more evenly throughout the body and are a great way to recruit satellite muscles so that mechanical damage to the muscles themselves is more evenly distributed.

All three forms of exercise are a great way to reduce inflammation in the body and improve overall health and longevity.

How do we reduce stress?

Exercise on its own is a form of stress-reduction strategy. So much so, as a matter of fact, that a meta-analysis of more than 200 research papers on the subject reached the conclusion that the effectiveness of exercise as a treatment for depression is so convincing that it should be prescribed just like any medicine.

The World Health Organization (WHO) defines stress as "a state of worry or mental tension caused by a difficult situation." It goes on to say that it is a natural human response that helps us address challenges and threats in our lives.

Stress releases adrenaline in our body and cortisol. Cortisol regulates the way our metabolic system uses glucose and plays a role in the way glycogen is synthesized in the liver and broken down in skeletal muscle.

In the ancient past where our bodies were forged this was an amazing way to elevate physical and mental preparedness, face a threat and remain systematically alert until it had passed and then recover.

In the modern world where we live we get to experience all the processes that prepare us to face the challenges and threats of modern living with none of the actual release. Because we no longer have to run, jump or fight the neurochemicals that stimulate us remain bottled up in our system and they are killing us.

The American Institute of Stress reports 120,000 people die every year as a direct result of work-related stress and the U.S. Department of Justice, in its Virtual Library that houses over 235,000 criminal justice resources, has an article with the heading: "Stress is the No 1 Killer" within their profession. In it, it cites how stress leads to asthma, heart attacks, high blood pressure and ulcers as well as drug and other substance abuse.

Stress then is a definitive problem. One that exercise can resolve quickly, inexpensively and, because regular exercise changes us physically and mentally, permanently.

Other physical interventions we can apply to help resolve it are: breathing and meditation. There are numerous studies on the ability of both to change blood chemistry and brain physiology which means that they are two relatively simple ways anyone can employ to re-establish their inner balance, reduce stress and feel more in control of their life.

How Food Can Fight Inflammation In The Body

Anything that relieves or reduces stress helps reduce the degree of inflammation experienced by organs and other tissues inside the body. When there is reduced inflammation the body has more resources at its disposal to do everything that is necessary for its upkeep. We feel stronger and healthier.

We've always been told that food provides the fundamental nutrients necessary for the body to run correctly. So, could we use food as one more means of intervention in our internal world to help ourselves feel better?

There are indeed hundreds if not thousands of food stuffs that range from herbs to specific natural food items that combat inflammation in the body. But over-indulging in them is never a good idea. Our uniqueness as individuals is never more pronounced than when we look at the populations of bacteria present in our gut that help us digest the food we eat.

Collectively called the microbiome, this population of gut bacteria also plays a role in mood, cognition and immune system health. Its uniqueness in each individual also makes it hard to be prescriptive in a one-size-fits-all diet. Everyone reacts to food differently and every microbiome processes food differently. So while, in principle, we all have the same nutritional needs, how we get them will vary from one individual to another.

Having said that, an anti-inflammatory diet is not that hard to figure out. It is any diet that includes a variety of plant-based foods and fiber, cuts down on excessive fat, salt and sugar and reduces the amount of processed foods and red meat consumed.

The goal here is not to apply a particular diet like keto, the Mediterranean diet, vegetarian or vegan. These are options that may not work for everyone. Instead it is much better for your mental and physical health to focus on eating food that has as few side-effects as possible and provides your body with all the nutrients it needs.

If you apply that principle in what you eat, you're giving yourself the best chance possible to stay healthy and feel strong.

It doesn't take a degree in medical science to connect the food we put inside our body with the effects it has on its tissues at a cellular level. Just because something is obvious however doesn't mean we automatically know how to make best use of it. When it comes to choosing what to eat, each day, we are governed by what is easily available, affordable and tasty. Unfortunately this is not always the best recipe for long-term health.

The World Health Organization (WHO) report on health highlights that worldwide 650 million adults, 340 million adolescents and 39 million children suffer from obesity. That's over 1 billion people who suffer from a condition that directly impacts their quality of life, impairs their health, affects their mental health and shortens their lifespan.

It shouldn't take a degree in food science to learn what foods work better for us and how to avoid the ones that don't help us much.

Here's what we need to get from the food we eat:

- Fiber
- Energy
- Nutrients

Here's what the food we eat should do for us:

- Reduce the inflammation in our body.
- Build our muscles and repair our tissues.

- Help us feel mentally and emotionally good.

So it's fair to say that the food we eat is fuel for our body and brain and while it fuels us it should also make it easier for us to function by reducing inflammation in our tissue. What food choices you make depend on the amount of money you have to spend on food each week, where you are geographically, what is available to you in your region and what support you have from your family and friends.

An anti-inflammatory diet is designed to do two things: First, give you some idea of what food choices to make in order to reduce and repair chronic inflammation in your body. Second, what food choices to make in order to avoid causing inflammation in your body in the first instance.

The guidelines are fairly simple:

Eat more fruit and vegetables to add more fiber to your diet. Vary your diet according to what is produced locally and is available seasonally. Add omega-3 fatty acid rich food to your choice. Good sources of omega-3, which is known for its anti-inflammatory effects, are tofu, walnuts, soybeans, flux seeds, salmon and tuna. There are strong anti-inflammatory substances found in foods such as blueberries, garlic, olive oil, tea, celery, grapes and certain spices such as tumeric, ginger and rosemary.

Generally look for whole foods. Brown rice and whole wheat bread are great examples.

Reduce inflammatory foods such as white flour, white rice, refined sugar, red meat, deep fried and processed foods and anything with corn oil or margarine.

If you have never tried cooking and eating anything that isn't highly processed you now face a little bit of a learning curve. While you're learning I would suggest you just do this in the first instance: cut out anything that is high in sugar and anything that is highly processed. No fast food or, at the very least reduce the amount of fast food you eat. No sausages. No desserts after food (allow yourself to enjoy these only on the weekends). No white, sliced bread. No bacon. (I know, but trust me, this will help you).

Monitor how you feel in your new way of eating. Double-down on foods that help you feel strong and be healthy.

The Stress Response

We need stress to survive. Each morning we wake up because the cortisol levels in our bloodstream begin to rise. Cortisol is a stress hormone that increases our heartbeat, raises the temperature in our muscles and prepares us for action during our waking time.

It's not stress that's bad for us. It's unmanageable stress that's bad for us. Imagine stress as steam in a steam train. The role of Cortisol here is played by coal which is fed to a furnace by a boilerman. The boilerman's job is to shovel coal in the furnace that heats up the water that drives the steam that powers the steam engine.

As long as the steam engine does the work necessary to move the train, the steam that is produced by the fire in the furnace that is being fed coal by the boilerman is a good thing. The more coal that is being fed the higher the fire in the furnace burns and the more steam is produced and the more work is being done by the steam engine.

Imagine now that the steam engine is idle. What should happen here is that the boilerman has to take a welcome break and stop shoveling coal in the furnace. But what if he doesn't? What if no one told the boilerman that he can legitimately take a break? Then the furnace will keep on burning high and steam will continue to be produced but without an outlet that steam only keeps building up until it reaches critical level, exceeds the tolerance of the steam dome where it is stored which, in turn, explodes. That is the end of the steam engine.

Now imagine that instead of coal we use Cortisol and instead of steam we use stress and instead of the steam dome we use our organs. Without an outlet stress just keeps building up and as it builds up it exceeds our tolerance. Unlike a steam engine however we don't explode. But we do malfunction.

Stress causes our cells to misuse energy and even handle food incorrectly so that we can put on weight even if we don't necessarily overeat.

The body's Stress Response (which is what the Cortisol effect really is) is yet another ancient mechanism designed to help us survive by building up a good head of steam quickly so we can take action.

When we are faced with the prospect of a saber tooth tiger we need to run from or kill, an opposing tribe we have to deal with or a natural disaster we need to escape from, the rapidly rising Cortisol levels in our bloodstream are a benefit. In a modern office or home environment however, not so much.

So, we're left with building that head of steam in our engine without an outlet or safety valve. It's no wonder things begin to go physically and mentally wrong for us after some time spent exposed to chronic stress.

How do we deal with that? What interventions can we put in place that will help us "take the edge off" so we can function? And by interventions we are talking about practical things we can do that do not involve taking medicine, drinking alcohol, smoking or indulging in psychoactive substances that ultimately harm us.

Obviously, there is exercise. Walking, running, lifting, dancing and stretching are great ways to decompress the body, recharge the mind and get rid of the stress that has built up inside us. Studies have repeatedly shown that regular exercise builds emotional resilience that makes it easier for us to manage the stress we encounter. But until we actually get to the point where exercise is our safety valve how do we start to deal with stress better?

Plus, how do we deal with stress in situations where we can't just take off and go and do some exercise?

This is where breathing enters the picture. If we don't breathe we will die. The breathing reflex is something so deeply ingrained in us that we barely give it a thought. It is something that we think we are already really good at simply because we are alive.

It's not true. Sure, we all breathe. But just because we all breathe doesn't mean we do it right. Consider the physical symptoms of fear and anxiety: a tightness in the chest and stomach, a short and shallow breathing pattern and, if we were to wire up some monitoring equipment at the time, we would also notice increased skin electro-conductivity, and clamminess.

Prolonged stress reduces the amount of oxygen that is present in our bloodstream which then affects the health of all internal organs including the brain and impairs the way muscles function.

To better understand how something as simple as breathing can reduce the amount of stress we experience in situations and circumstances we don't control we need to take a bird's eye view of the body's nervous system and its components.

Without oversimplifying matters consider that the nervous system is divided into two key subsystems: the central nervous system (CNS) and the peripheral nervous system (PNS). The brain and spinal cord are the central nervous system and the vast network of nerves radiating from the spine is the peripheral nervous system. It helps to think of the central nervous system as the central telephone exchange, the center where all the computers are and the peripheral nervous system as the cabling that runs across a city connecting all the different masts, towers and buildings.

A component of the peripheral nervous system is the autonomic nervous system. Its function is to control our internal organs and glands and it is called 'autonomic' because we don't have conscious control of it.

The autonomic nervous system in turn is divided into three anatomically distinct divisions called the sympathetic nervous system, the parasympathetic nervous system and the enteric nervous system. Despite the name the sympathetic and parasympathetic nervous systems have nothing to do with sympathy.

These two systems control the same parts of the body and the same general functions but each has an opposite effect to the other. The sympathetic nervous system raises the alarm throughout the body by dialing up our stress responses to better prepare us for physical action (the traditional "fight or flight" response). The parasympathetic nervous system works to return our internal chemistry and the state of our internal organs back to what it was before the alarm was raised. It is the calming down agent.

So far we appear to be a network of connections that run in parallel to each other but are distinct. This, however is not how we function at all. The enteric nervous system that runs digestion and secretes specific hormones, is connected to the central nervous system by the longest nerve in our body which originates in the brain stem and ends its connection in our large intestine. This is called the vagus nerve, more popularly referred to as 'the brain/gut axis' or 'the brain/gut connection' and it is part of the parasympathetic nervous system (that controls involuntary processes including breathing).

If you've ever been punched hard in the solar plexus you know that terrible feeling where you double up and can't breathe. A blow that should only hurt us with a little bit of physical pain can actually disrupt the involuntary signals the brain sends to our diaphragm through the vagus nerve and interfere with the signaling of the brain that enables our lungs to expand and compress so we can inhale and exhale.

Such is the disruption caused to our breathing, through impact on the vagus nerve, that a hard enough punch will disrupt it long enough for us to pass out.

Bridging Two Separate Systems

Think of a day when things get a little too much for you. What do you do? Chances are that at some point you will sigh. Neuroscience tells us that a sigh is a reflex action that is defined as a deep, long breath like an inhale and exhale but not quite like it.

The mechanics of sighing may be very similar to those of normal breathing because we only have one mechanical set up that helps us breathe. The action and its effect however are very different.

A sigh is the response of the part of the brain that closely monitors our stress levels. It has a dual role. If we are really stressed and our breathing is shallow and our chest muscles are constricted and our blood oxygen levels drop a sigh becomes a deep breath that tries to address this problem so that our alertness does not dip.

If, however, we have been stressed and we successfully powered our way through whatever it was that we had to do we are entitled to what we popularly call "a sigh of relief". Again, we breathe deep as we sigh, we replenish oxygen supplies in our bloodstream but the sigh, this time, activates a different part of our nervous system and powers our excited and hyper-alert state back to normal levels.

What happens when we sigh then is that we use our breathing apparatus to activate either the sympathetic nervous system (and raise our level of alertness) or activate our parasympathetic nervous system (and calm ourselves down).

We do both of these actions by stimulating the vagus nerve. The vagus nerve is the lock that activates or shuts down either of these two systems and the involuntary sighs we experience as well as more consciously directed breathing, are the key.

When we think about this in terms of our ancient past we understand it makes perfect sense. We need a stress response in order to survive. Depending on what we have to do: run, fight, climb and so on, deep breathing is in direct response to the physical exertion we engage in and it will activate the vagus nerve and will, during our time of need, give us all the oxygen and alertness we need to succeed in our task. After our exertions, deep breathing will again play a role in calming us down and bring our internal state back to its natural, balanced baseline.

Most problems we experience with stress in a modern setting are caused by the fact that we no longer have to hunt, run, jump or fight in order to get through our day. We sit, instead, behind a desk or, if we have a physically demanding job, have to perform relatively few tasks in a controlled manner.

We do not have the opportunity to get rid of the head of steam building up inside us. This is what we can do instead: Take a deep breath slowly until our lungs fill up to what we think is their full capacity. Hold it for a second. And then take one more breath on top of it. Hold that for another second or two and now slowly exhale.

This is called the double-sigh and it is an excellent way to stimulate the vagus nerve. The moment we do that we feel clear-headed, calm and ready for anything.

Take Action

Problem: None of us fully takes into account and tracks the type of physical activity required to keep us young and active or the correct combination of exercise, sleep and nutrition we need to keep us mentally and physically balanced. Nor does any of us try to quantify the amount of stress we are exposed to because of our lifestyle and our immediate environment.

Solution: Keep a detailed diary of your life. The things you do, the activities you engage in, what you experience and how these things make you feel. It is only by keeping track of the things we do and the things we experience that we can get to the stage where we know what to do more of and what we must try to decrease our exposure to or avoid altogether in order to maintain our mental and physical health.

Action Plan

Start a diary. Record your daily activities, nutrition and, if possible, experiences and feelings. If you think you can quantify, however subjectively, the amount of stress you feel each day from a scale of one to ten, do so. Try, when you record it, to also explain what you think caused all that stress (or lack of it). Work on your breathing by being consciously aware of how you breathe when, for instance, you experience stress and strive to take deeper, more relaxed breaths. Use breathing when stressed to calm yourself both internally and externally.

There are eight workouts that follow this chapter. They are, as always with DAREBEE workouts, extensively field-tested. They're designed to help your body feel better and your brain and mind recharge and rejuvenate. While every workout helps us change inside and out those that specifically target changes in our inner world are more restorative than others and these are good to have in your arsenal.

THE GUT

DAREBEE WORKOUT
© darebee.com

Level I   3 sets
Level II   5 sets
Level III 7 sets
2 minutes rest

10 march steps
10 high knees

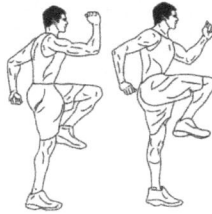

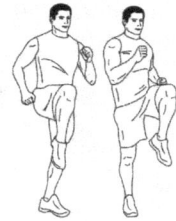

10 march steps
10 climbers

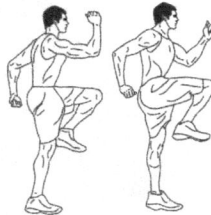

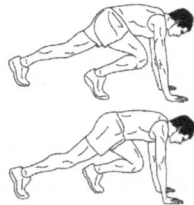

10 march steps
10 knee-to-elbow

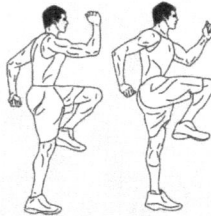

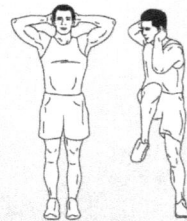

TIME
OF MY
LIFE

DAREBEE WORKOUT
© darebee.com
LEVEL I 3 sets
LEVEL II 5 sets
LEVEL III 7 sets
REST up to 2 minutes

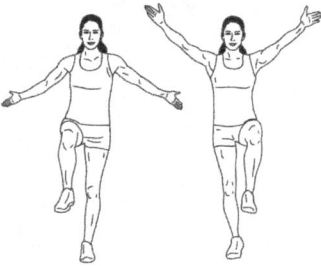

10 march with wide circles

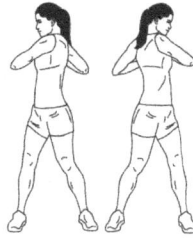

10 torso twists

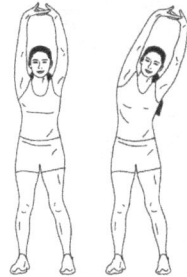

10 side bends

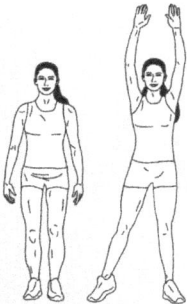

10 step jacks

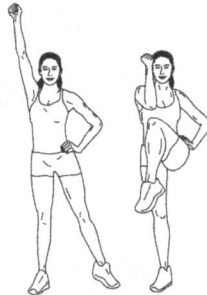

10 knee to elbows

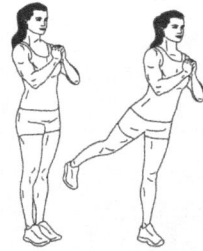

10 back leg raises

REAL

WORKOUT by DAREBEE © darebee.com
30 seconds rest between sets | No rest between exercises

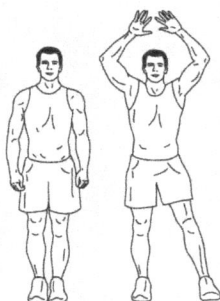

10 step jacks
x 3 sets in total

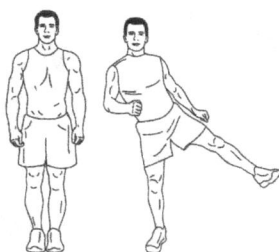

20 side leg raises
x 3 sets in total

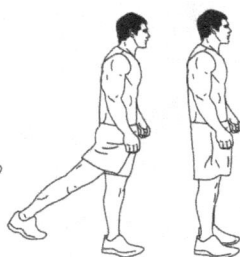

20 back leg raises
x 3 sets in total

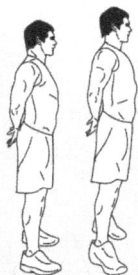

10 calf raises
x 3 sets in total

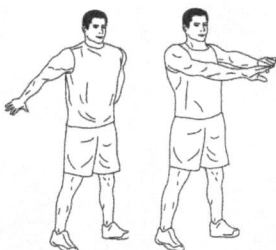

20 arm raises
x 3 sets in total

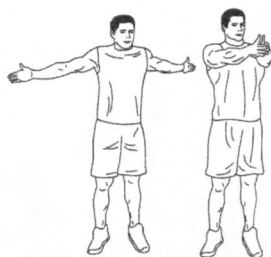

20 chest expansions
x 3 sets in total

reset
stretching

DAREBEE WORKOUT © darebee.com
Count to 10 while holding each stretch (for each side).

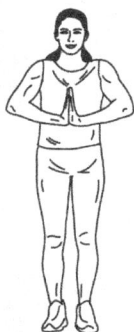

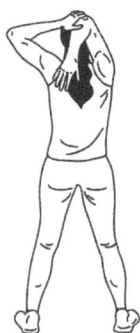

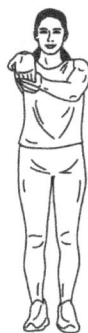

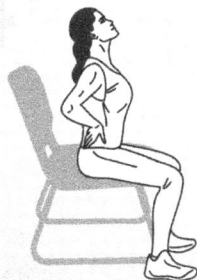

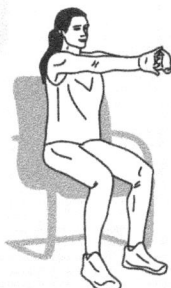

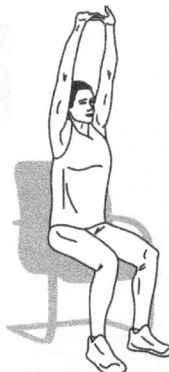

ZEN

DAREBEE WORKOUT © **darebee.com**
Hold each pose for 30 seconds then move on to the next one.

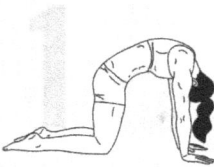

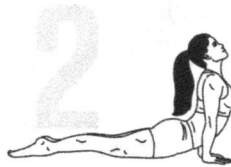

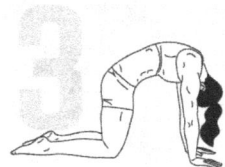

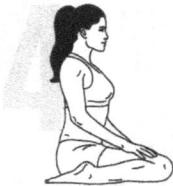

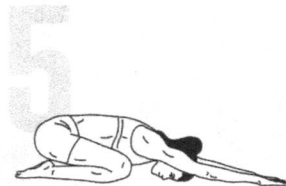

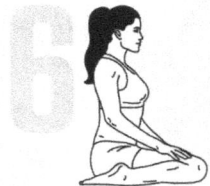

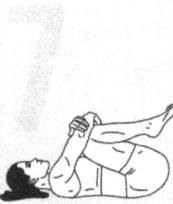

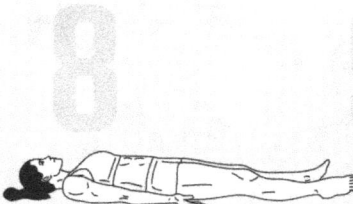

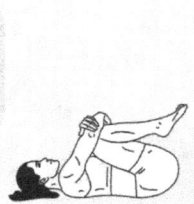

SITTING FIX

DAREBEE WORKOUT © darebee.com
Count to 10 while holding each stretch (for each side).

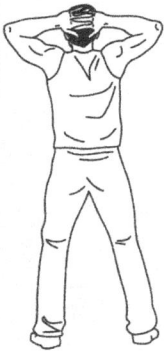

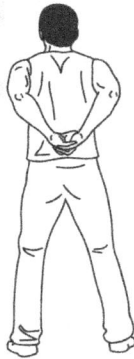

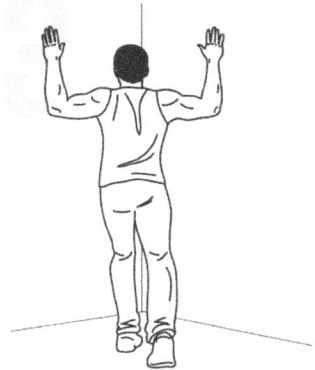

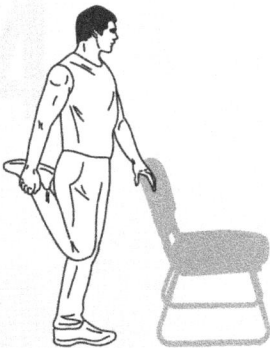

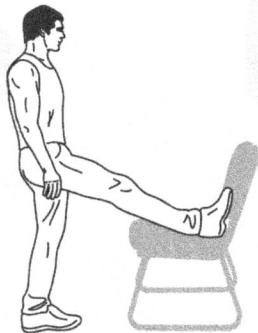

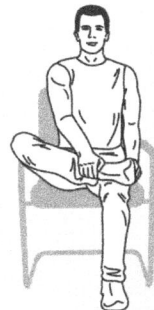

rawr

DAREBEE WORKOUT © darebee.com

Hold each pose for 30 seconds then move on to the next one.
Repeat the sequence again on the other side.

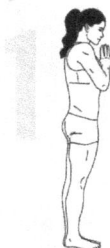

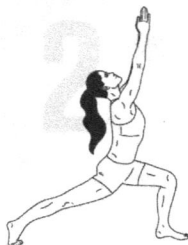

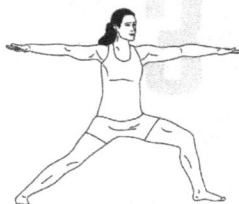

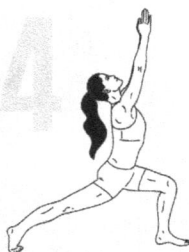

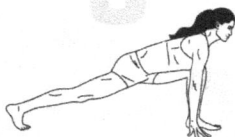

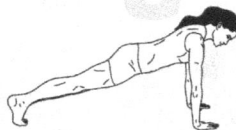

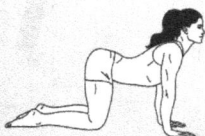

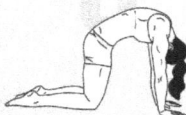

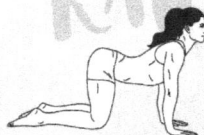

RAWR!

before BED

WORKOUT
BY DAREBEE
© darebee.com

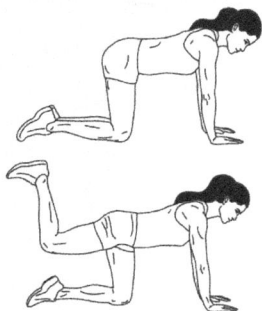

40 leg extensions

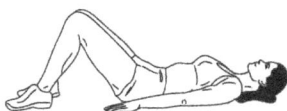

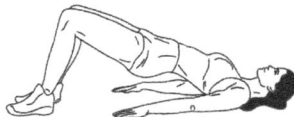

20 bridges

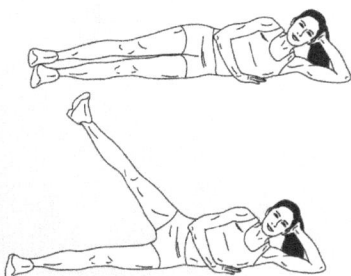

40 side leg raises

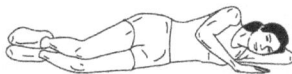

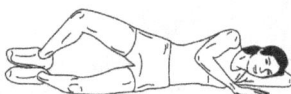

20 clamshells

The four field-tested DAREBEE workouts that follow are again, intended to help you re-center yourself, recharge and reset your inner balance. You can use them any time, anywhere but they are particularly useful when you are short on time.

harmony

DAREBEE WORKOUT © darebee.com

Hold each pose for 60 seconds then move on to the next one.

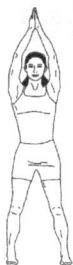

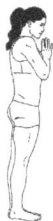

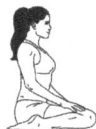

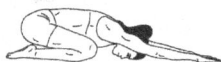

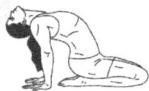

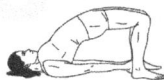

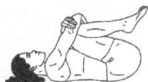

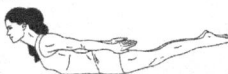

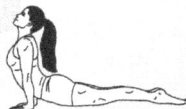

STRESS BUSTER

DAREBEE WORKOUT © darebee.com

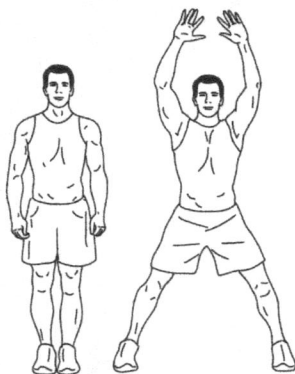

5 jumping jacks

5 chest expansions

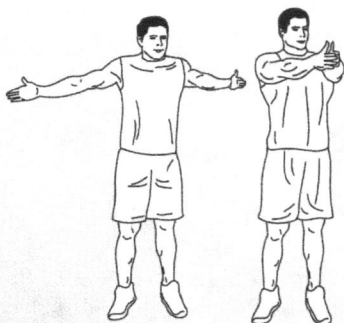

5 jumping jacks

5 chest expansions

5 jumping jacks

5 chest expansions

done

60-second
de-stress

by DAREBEE © **darebee.com** stretching
Repeat each one for 10 seconds.

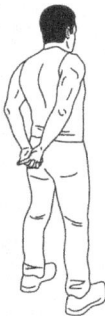
back stretch

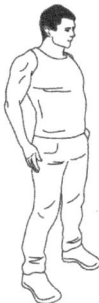
shoulder rotations

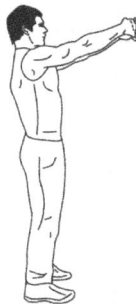
arm stretch

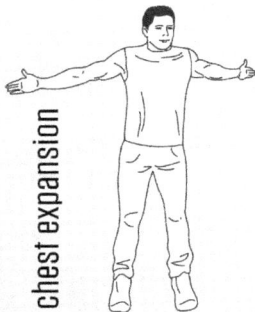
chest expansion

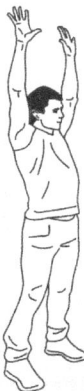
overhead reach

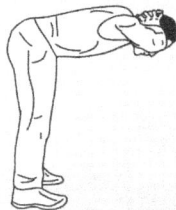
forward bend

breathe
easy

WORKOUT by © darebee.com

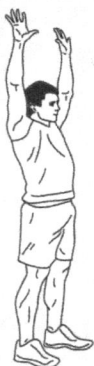

Arms above your head

1) Breathe in deep;
2) Hold to count of five;
3) Exhale to count of five.

Repeat 5 times in total.

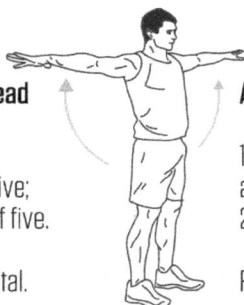

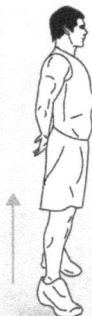

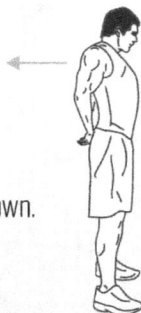

Arm Raises

1) Breathe in
as you raise your arms;
2) Exhale on the way down.

Repeat 5 times in total.

Calf Raises

1) Breathe in as you rise;
2) Hold to count of five;
3) Exhale as you drop down.

Repeat 5 times in total.

Shoulder Stretches
arms behind your back

1) Breathe in as you stretch;
2) Hold to count of five;
3) Exhale as you relax.

Repeat 5 times in total.

THE SECRET DRIVES

Beliefs are explanations. Values are priorities. Actions are a reflection of who we truly are. It is in the consistency of our actions that we manifest not just who we are but also who we want to become.

Why do you do anything you do? I'm not talking about getting up in the morning and going to work, we all have to do something like that in one form or another. I'm asking why do you do the things you want to do? Why do you go to the cinema? Why do you organize a trip out with friends? Why do you go to a football match? Why do you, if you do, get dressed and go to the gym on a cold winter evening?

The answer here (and it sounds a little like cheating) is motivation. I say it sounds like cheating because obviously every time you do something and it doesn't really matter what that is, you are neurochemically motivated to do it. If you weren't you wouldn't do it.

So what is motivation exactly? Neurobiology tells us that motivation is the feeling we experience when a particular group of neurotransmitters builds up to a certain level in our brain at which point a specific action is undertaken. But that is a very difficult picture to understand. We have no sense of these neurotransmitters building up inside us and we certainly do not feel the electrical impulses across synapses in our brain that move us to action.

We do however sense when things are not going well for us and we become disconcerted and disgruntled and uncomfortable. At some point the level of discomfort we experience reaches a point that exceeds our ability to tolerate it and that is when we are moved to action.

Motivation therefore is our moving from a point of discomfort to a point of comfort. The definition is the same whether the discomfort we feel is basic, as in thirst or hunger, physical as in pain or emotional as in anxiety and distress.

We review motivation in such broad strokes to highlight the fact that when we say we are not motivated to exercise or we have lost our motivation what we are actually saying is that the condition we are currently in is not yet bad enough for us to decide to do something about.

Of course when things do get bad enough for us to actually want to exercise we are in such poor physical shape that the job itself has become so much harder that just starting is overwhelming and an obstacle we must learn to overcome.

This is what I will say about our body: it is a gift. A temporary one at that. We have been given the extraordinary ability to move ourselves around the planet under our own power and experience the magic of the world through our senses.

If this body we each have was a borrowed one we'd owe it to the entity we borrowed it from to keep it in tip-top shape and give it back, when the term of our contract expired in the same pristine condition we received it. Much like we do with a car-hire contract actually.

While we all have a finite number of years on this planet our focus on the now stops us from considering that the time we have is not all that much and that we might even have a lot less time than we think we have due to circumstances beyond our control.

Do we really then want to deprive ourselves of all the possible experiences we can have with our body? Would we want to go through life and not be able to enjoy it and the world around us as fully as possible? Do we want to have a short life or one where its quality is so impaired that we wake up each day and struggle?

These are questions we need to ask ourselves and then answer them as honestly as we can. It is only in the honesty of our answers that we should expect to find the motivation we think we lack to be the best physical and mental versions of ourselves possible.

Note that this is not a competition, nor should it be one. It's not about being the strongest or the fastest or the fittest by whatever measure we care to measure being strong, fast or fit by. It is, instead, about feeling capable in our own body. It is about going through life and feeling that we are capable of dealing with anything that comes up because our body is under our control and our brain and mind are ours, also.

The Paradox Of Motivation

In the very first chapter of this book we saw how when it comes to fitness no one has a clear idea of what it actually should be. What we form is what is given to us by the external world and other people's expectations, perceptions, ideas and thoughts based on what is important to them.

No one, really, stops to consider what is right for us. What we might want to achieve when it comes to fitness. We therefore start a love/hate relationship with fitness and exercise that seesaws between what is expected of us, what we think is expected of us and how we think we are perceived by those who we think expect something from us.

It's a brain twister, I know. That's what makes it hard. That's why we don't sometimes exercise - because we're afraid of being judged and found wanting. That's why we put off doing what is right for us - because we are not sure if it fits in with what everyone else thinks we should be doing.

In discussions with friends I have often have them tell me "I need to start exercising a little so I can get fitter for the gym" like the gym is a place with some kind of minimum fitness requirement for entry. Yet, when you truly think about it a gym is often seen as a place where fit people go to become even fitter.

The idea of barely clothed bodies on show has us thinking that we must have already attained some kind of basic standard of perceived physical beauty in order to just be there.

Our society is a little screwed up about things like that. But there is hope.

We are slowly (and I do mean slowly) beginning to reconsider what it is to be fit. We are beginning to understand that when it comes to fitness, balance and happiness are more important than a lean body mass, a precisely regulated diet and the ability to exhibit athleticism.

The same goes for motivation.

I am sure, you will come across people who think that motivation is something that somehow just runs out suddenly, like a consumable. Or it is something they need to find. Or it is something that other people have more of. None of this is true.

We are motivated by emotions, not thoughts. Just thinking doesn't work and we know it. We all see the disheartening drop-out figures of people who make a resolution to go to the gym in January and have dropped out completely by mid-February. We have all seen the incredible figures of the number of people who don't exercise and the scary figures of the number of people who suffer or will suffer from obesity and its attendant health problems.

The problem we have with motivation and exercise stems from the disconnect between the things we know and the things we feel. Right now we feel OK. Our emotions are mostly balanced, our inner state is relatively stable. The reason we know we need to exercise is in the future and although we all know that we will get old, we all know that physically and mentally we will change and degrade, we all know that emotionally we will be in a much worse state in that future, we don't feel it. Most of us have a really hard time imagining how we shall feel if we are physically slower, or if our mobility is severely restricted, or if our health has been impacted so we can no longer enjoy the things we enjoy doing.

For sure we will be motivated to act the moment we feel those things, but because that moment lies in the future we fail to take action in the present. We simply cannot imagine, in the present moment, just how bad we will feel if we allow ourselves to become ill, or if we allow ourselves to become old.

We cannot imagine how the happiness we feel in the present will become harder for us to feel in the future if we are not healthy and strong.

That is the paradox of motivation. That is the explanation why so many of us don't feel sufficiently motivated to exercise. And we've already seen all the other internal and external obstacles we face when it comes to exercise.

Our civilization is, by most accounts, about 6,000 years old. In that time we have managed to mostly remove most physical threats to us and have ensured, again mostly, that no matter where we are on the planet we can enjoy a sense of physical security. No one is going to come and kill us for our possessions or our food or the clothes we wear.

I understand this is a relative achievement and there are some factors that contribute to it that are not yet universal but by and large it is true and it is a magnificent achievement. At the same time no one yet looks out for our physical health or our mental health or our general well-being. We do not yet have rules and regulations in place regarding being nice to people or being considerate or thinking about their well-being as well as ours.

We do not yet really have unwritten societal rules that guide public behavior which would safeguard our mental health and help us avoid ruinous mistakes that would destroy our physical and mental balance. Again, there are some exceptions to this, but as a generalization, this observation is mostly and sadly, still true.

At some point, I expect, we will get there. The body positivity movement that tries to remove judgment, the open talk about mental health issues we all see on social media, the various projects around the planet such as the good men project that examine gender behavior and actively encourage inclusivity and the many other similar movements that are taking off all the time, are encouraging signs that we are still evolving our thinking and refining our approach.

It brings me now to the nitty-gritty. How to use all this so that you, as an individual, can stand out from your peers by your ability to understand that the future you is a direct result of the investment of effort you put in your present self.

Run this exercise: Sit down and consider how you want yourself to be five years from now. Write down your age and weight. Write down what you think your athletic ability will be. Be specific. If you can run 100m in 20 seconds now extrapolate from your current knowledge of yourself and project what that will be like five years from your present. Then, if you can, write down also what you would like it to be if you had all the time and money in the world.

Write down all the other specifics: where do you see yourself living. With whom? Doing what? Create a granular but reasonable picture of the future you as you want it to be. Now consider what will it take to make that picture real?

Don't cheat yourself here by placing an insurmountable obstacle. Don't say, for instance, "a million dollars" because you imagine that if you had all that money and the leisure it could afford you, you would be able to become the person you imagine. Be realistic. Actually break down the steps that are truly required to help you become the person you imagine in your future.

If, for instance, you want the five-years-older you to be able to continue doing the 100m sprint in 20 seconds or even improve on that time, then define clearly and in detail the training you think is needed and the frequency in that training, required to make this happen.

Allow this exercise to consume you completely. Become immersed in the specifics like you are a reporter delivering a descriptive report from the future to yourself. When you have finished take a look at what you have written and for every chain of actions required to make something specific happen in that near future, ask yourself this question: what is stopping me?

Define the barriers you see with the same attention to detail you have given to everything else in this exercise. And now that you see each barrier in detail, come up with a workable solution that will remove it or circumvent it completely.

If, for example, you need access to a sprint track to help improve your sprinting and there simply isn't one where you are what acceptable substitution can you find? If you need a set of good quality weights and there simply are none to have or no means to get them, what can you do to get past that and substitute something that will give you the same results?

Do this for every requirement needed to make the future you happen. And when you are done, ask yourself one final question: When can you start your journey to become this future you?

Happiness

Everyone deserves to be happy. It's a little strange to look for happiness through exercise but scientifically it's a sound concept. I will explain it in a moment but let's start with yet another thought experiment I want you to participate in.

Let me take you into a purpose-built room. This room lies at the heart of an onion-like complex six layers thick, each layer is 12 inches of solid concrete. The room rests on 68 vibration-dampening springs which rest, in turn, on their own separate foundation slab. This room is so quiet that if you stand absolutely still you will be able to hear the sound of your own blood rushing through your arteries and, as you move, you will be able to hear your bones grinding as your joints move.

This room actually exists in the heart of Building 87 at Microsoft's Redmond Headquarters in Washington. It is part of the software giant's Orfield Labs and in 2015 it officially broke the Guinness World record for the quietest place on Earth.

Microsoft uses it to test the sound of electronic equipment it makes but its value to us, right now, lies in the effect it has on human visitors. Divorced from the constant pressure of air on their ears that they are used to in the world outside this room, most people report feeling disorientated, spooked, some even get dizzy. Staying in there for more than a few minutes becomes an uncomfortable experience.

You'd think that being in such a quiet place would be an opportunity for self-reflection perhaps, certainly a chance to feel liberated from the outside world and its constant demands on our attention but this is not the case.

The reason this truly impressively quiet room is so physically and mentally disconcerting to us, lies in the way we are constructed. Our body is a network of sensors constantly sampling our environment and our brain is a repository of knowledge, memories and experience through which are filtered all the signals from the outside world that our body reports.

Our emotions are created by the way our brain interprets the signals it receives from our body once it filters them through what we know and what we remember from what we've learned. The moment we remove the external world from our senses we've also removed a large chunk of how we feel inside ourselves.

Microsoft's quietest room on Earth feels wrong to us because without us realizing it, it cuts us off from a massive chunk of information the external world feeds to our brain through the senses of our body. All of which, of course, now brings us to happiness.

We all long so much to be happy that, according to a McKinsey report globally we spend $1.5 trillion a year trying to capture it, experience it or discover it. What does all this expensive activity we engage in as we pursue happiness have to do with exercise?

I'm going to unpack all of this for you now.

In English, the origin of the word emotion dates back to the 17th century as the adoption of the French word émotion which meant "physical disturbance" or "movement". The psychologist Dr. George W. Crane in his famous book Applied Psychology admonished his readers: "Remember, motions are the precursors of emotions. You can't control the latter directly but only through your choice of motions or actions."

Neuroscience views emotions as brief moments of coordinated brain, autonomic, and behavioral changes that facilitate a response to an event. The coordinated activity that takes place is founded in the change of a neurochemical state which is represented by specific neurobiological conditions. The response that is facilitated by all this is designed to, usually, return our internal world to its balanced, neutral state.

Emotions then are excitations. Something inside us is agitated and once that internal agitation reaches a specific internal threshold we are prompted to take action. If this sounds a little like the trigger we call "motivation" it's because from a neurobiological perspective that is exactly what it is.

But if emotion is what we feel because of an internal imbalance in our neurochemical states what prompts that imbalance in the first instance? The answer to that is a stimulus. Every stimulus we experience comes from the outside world. Every stimulus we experience needs to be processed and its processing creates, as a by-product, a neurochemical imbalance within us (let's call that an agitation). Depending on the assessment we then make the imbalance created by a stimulus may start a cascade of further imbalances (think of what happens when we hear a fire alarm go off in our building and you get the idea).

Each imbalance in sequence is followed by an effect and they all ultimately lead to an action. The action, in turn, satisfies the process or the sequence of processes that initiated it and leads us back to a state of balance.

Motion is movement, movement is emotion. Where does happiness come into it all?

Consider that every action is a movement that has an emotion as its point of origin. We initiate the action in order to go from a place where we felt agitated to a place where we feel at peace. The transition is happiness.

Remember that fire alarm in your building going off? You get agitated. The fire drill calls for you to evacuate via an approved route. You engage in that action because you understand that there is a risk of you getting burnt alive if you don't. You get outside the building and gather at an approved point to wait for the emergency situation to be over. The moment you are safely outside and at the approved point you basically chill. Whatever anxiety you experienced is over. You may not totally be aware of it but you are happy because you are safe.

When we exercise we basically introduce a stressor in our life that alters our internal states and changes our neurochemical make up. There are a whole lot of other complexities involved in this but we can safely ignore them for now. When the exercise period is over we settle down into a new state of internal balance that has the additional benefit of our having a higher blood oxygen level than usual and we feel at peace with ourselves and the world.

The more intensely we exercise the more acutely we feel that after-effect, which is why exercise in itself can become addictive. Happiness is that sense of peace and inner balance. It is the sense of self-worth we have when we have physically engaged in something that has tested us and have come out the other side.

When we experience stressors like exercise we are essentially teaching our brain and body to cope better with stressors in general. By moving our body we learn to become mentally and psychologically more resilient. And by becoming more resilient we are building up the mental and psychological equivalent of muscles.

The thing to remember is that happiness is a process we experience not a state we consume. We are happiest when we are in the process of becoming. We feel our best when we've been tested and have successfully come through the test.

Even the smallest of commitments like going for a walk in the early morning or evening, moving our body and letting our senses take in our surrounding world is enough to contribute towards a state of happiness.

The idea that we can use our body to make ourselves happier is given further backing by research led by cognitive scientist John Bargh at Yale University which shows that people who held a warm cup of coffee before a job interview found the individuals they talked afterwards warmer and kinder.

At the department of psychology at Michigan University Joshua Ackerman has shown through his research that the softness of the seat people seat on affects their decision making with negotiators becoming really difficult when they were sat on hard seats.

All of these are examples of embodied cognition more about which we shall discuss in the next chapter's section that looks at ways we can enjoy a healthy life for as long as possible. Embodied Cognition is the idea that the sensations of the body are essential for us to understand the world, create meaningful inferences and construct conceptual knowledge about it.

We think and feel, in other words, not with our brain and body but with the world and what we do with our brain and body in the world affects their internal states so that our thoughts, feelings and inclinations changes with our actions and the environment we are in.

Blue spaces, the broad name used to describe bodies of water such as lakes, streams, ponds and the sea, invariably raise the sense of happiness and well-being more than any other natural space. This has been highlighted in research published by Matthew White of the University of Vienna where he was able to quantify that research subjects exposed to blue spaces felt as proportionally happier as people who had left doing household chores to go out and socialize with friends.

Walking has been found to help lift even the darkest of moods and fresh research shows that it also increases cognition by activating the processing centers of the brain that are involved in strategic planning and factual analysis. Neurotransmitters released by walking include endorphins, endocannabinoids, and dopamine.

Does all this mean that just need exercise to make us happy? No, that is not what I've said here. Exercise, physical movement primarily, is the tool we use to rebalance our inner state. Happiness is the process we experience as that rebalancing takes place.

So exercise helps us to reach a state of happiness but it doesn't in itself make us happy. For that we need to strive, set goals, take action and go through the process necessary to reach the goals we have set and experience a physical (or virtual) environment that is diverse and contains as many natural elements as possible.

By engaging in physical activity we become more receptive to being happy. Accounts from Olympic medal winners who trained hard for many years to win in their sport at the highest level possible agree, that happiness in their post-athletic careers begins with happiness in their life, the choices they make and the way they live. And that becomes the foundation for better health after they stop competing.

Take Action

Problem: Our focus on the future makes us miss the present. Our struggle in the present absorbs so much of our energy we fail to truly imagine the future we want. Because we can't decide what to focus on and when we end up falling in the gap between the two.

Solution: Have a real talk with yourself. No, truly. Sit down, find a little quiet time and write down how you want your future life to be. How healthy and strong do you really want to be. How happy do you want to feel? Unless you articulate something it remains an unrealized possibility full of potential but of no actual value.

Action Plan

Unless you engage with your thoughts, hopes and ideas in a meaningful, concrete way they will forever remain potential things that might happen but most likely never do.

Make yourself accountable. Share your hopes and dreams with others. Listen to theirs. Surround yourself with people who are also striving to keep themselves accountable and real.

Integrate this plan of your fitness journey (both mental and physical) with your socializing goals and your plans to improve who you are physically and mentally, that way you are more likely to be consistent in your actions and also will not overburden yourself with activities and feel the 'burn out' that happens when you do too much and get less back than you expected.

Keeping a diary or a journal is a powerful aid in this regard. It creates a powerful outlet for those moments when life gets overwhelming and we may find ourselves with no immediate person to share our burdens with and it becomes a useful aid when we plan the path that takes us from the present to the future.

The following eight DAREBEE workouts are mood-changers. If you're feeling low, if you want a mood-boost, if you want to feel your body move and your mood change then these eight, field-tested workouts are just for you.

Happy Hour

DAREBEE WORKOUT © darebee.com
10 sets with 2 minute rest between sets
20 seconds each exercise

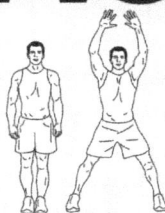

2 minutes
jumping jacks
pre workout
warmup

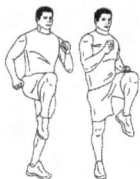

high knees

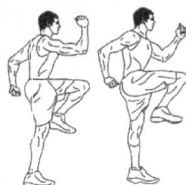

march steps

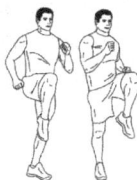

high knees

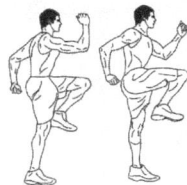

march steps

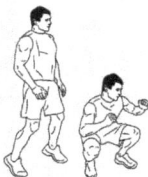

squats

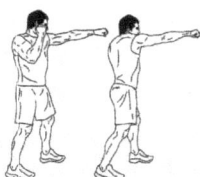

punches

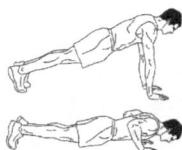

push-ups

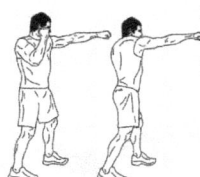

punches

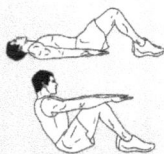

sit-ups

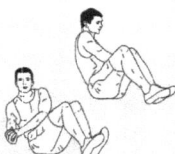

sitting twists

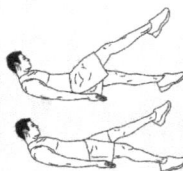

flutter kicks

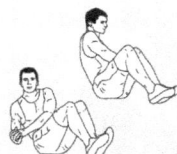

sitting twists

feel**good**

DAREBEE WORKOUT © darebee.com

LEVEL I 3 sets **LEVEL II** 4 sets **LEVEL III** 5 sets **REST** up to 2 minutes

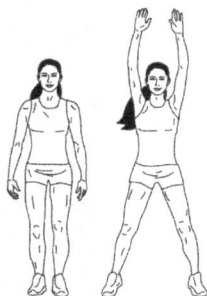

10 jumping jacks

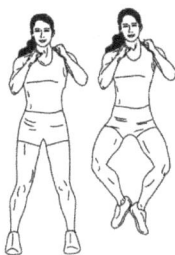

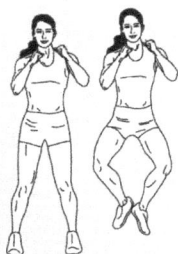

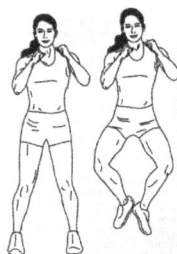

2 hop heel clicks

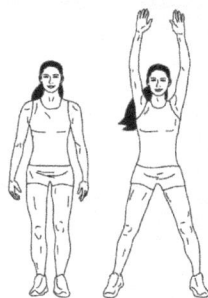

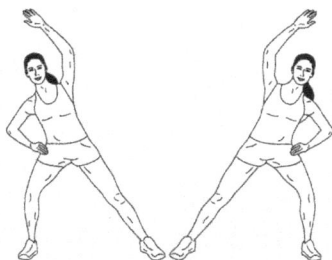

10 jumping jacks

2 hop heel clicks

10 side jacks

2 hop heel clicks

FEEL GOOD NOW

DAREBEE WORKOUT
© darebee.com
LEVEL I 3 sets
LEVEL II 5 sets
LEVEL III 7 sets
REST up to 2 minutes

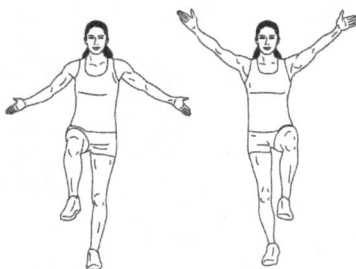

20 march steps with arm circles

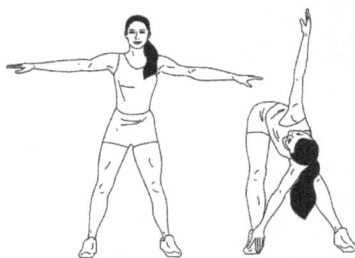

20 windmills

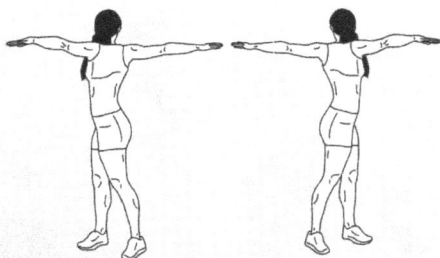

20 raised arms twists

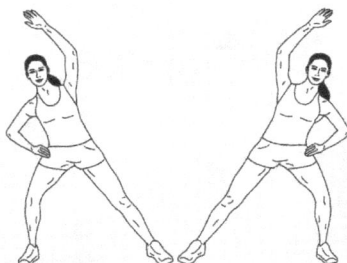

20 side jacks

That's How I
CELEBRATE

DAREBEE WORKOUT © darebee.com

LEVEL I 3 sets **LEVEL II** 5 sets **LEVEL III** 7 sets **REST** up to 2 minutes

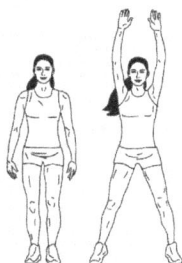

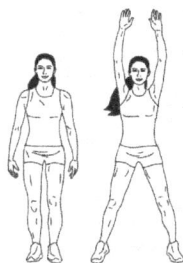

12 jumping jacks

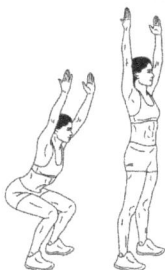

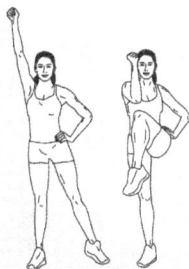

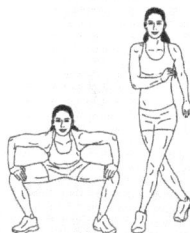

6 high squats

12 jumping jacks

6 knee to elbow

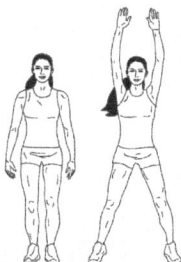

12 jumping jacks

6 squat step back

Good Day

DAREBEE WORKOUT
© darebee.com
LEVEL I 3 sets
LEVEL II 5 sets
LEVEL III 7 sets
REST up to 2 minutes

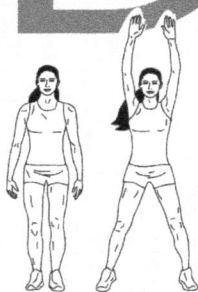

10 jumping jacks

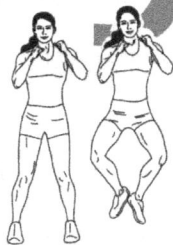

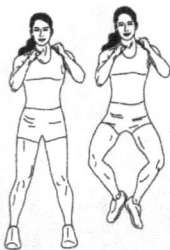

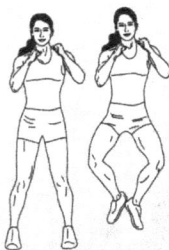

one hop heel click

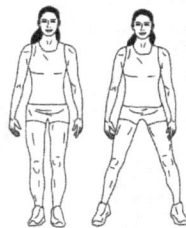

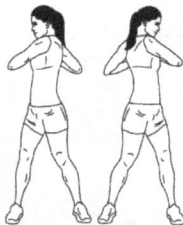

10 half jacks

one hop heel click

10 twists

one hop heel click

feel alive

DAREBEE WORKOUT © darebee.com

LEVEL I 3 sets **LEVEL II** 5 sets **LEVEL III** 7 sets **REST** up to 2 minutes

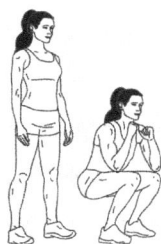

10 squats

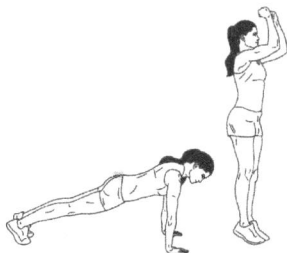

5 basic burpees

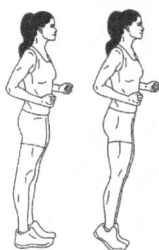

10 calf raises

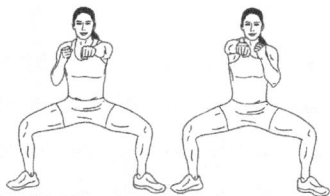

20 squat hold punches

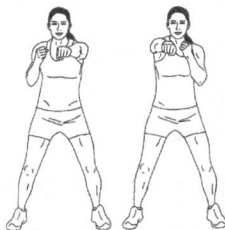

20 punches

Setting Goals

WORKOUT
BY DAREBEE
© darebee.co[m]

Level I 3 sets
Level II 5 sets
Level III 7 sets
2 minutes rest

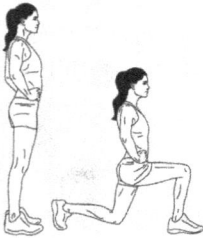

4 lunges

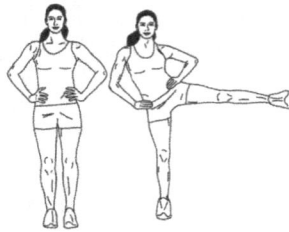

20 side leg raises

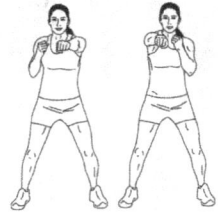

20 punches

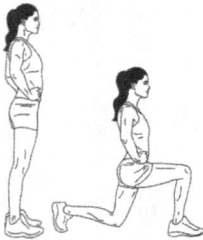

4 lunges

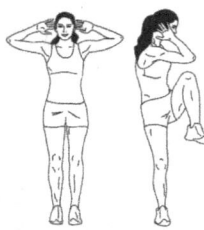

4 knee-to-elbows

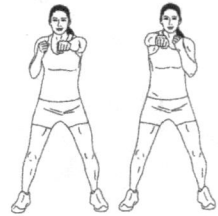

20 punches

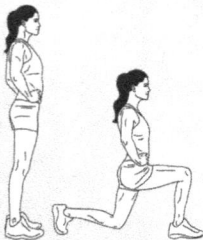

4 lunges

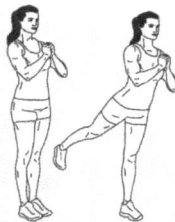

20 back leg raises

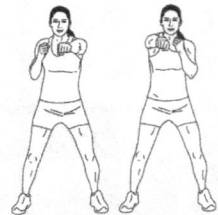

20 punches

WAKE UP!
& MAKE IT HAPPEN

DAREBEE WORKOUT © darebee.com

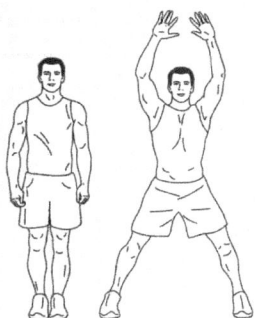 **20** jumping jacks

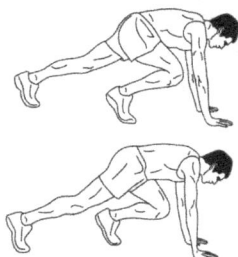 **20** climbers

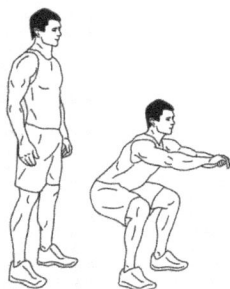 **20** squats

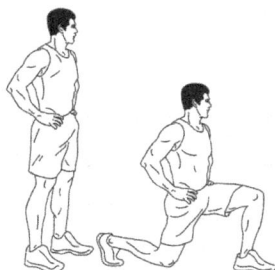 **20** lunges

20 push-ups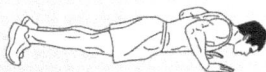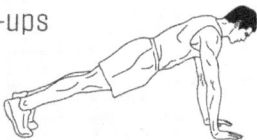

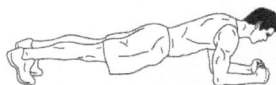 **20-count** elbow plank hold

Crunched for time? Not sure what you can do? Then these four, quick DAREBEE workouts are just what you need to help keep your body revving until you find the time and energy for something a little bit more intensive. As an added bonus they can be used to supplement whatever else you're doing so that you can make fitness gains even when you're not actively spending a lot of time working out.

HAPPY FEET

DAREBEE WORKOUT © darebee.com
20 seconds each

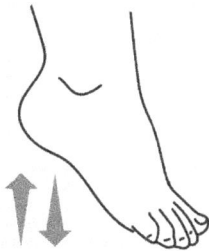

1. floor taps

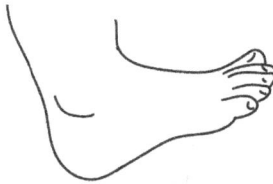

2. raise and hold

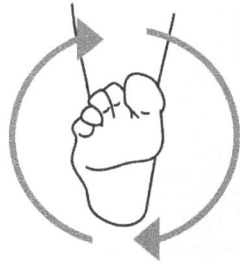

3. rotations

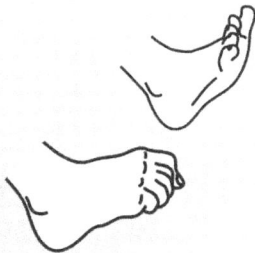

4. clench / unclench

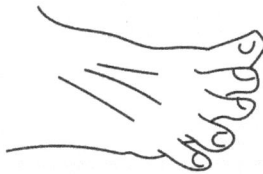

5. toes spread & hold

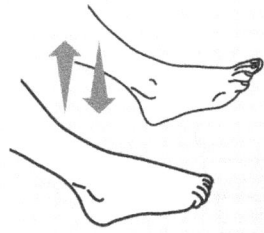

6. shake!

my HAPPY PLACE

WORKOUT
BY DAREBEE
© darebee.com

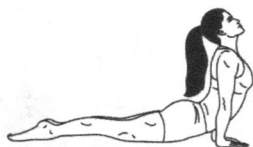

60sec stretch #1

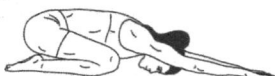

60sec stretch #2

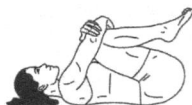

60sec stretch #3

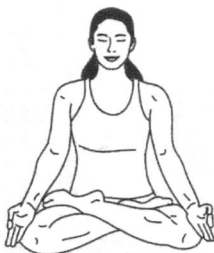

10 minutes meditation

2-minute abs

DAREBEE WORKOUT © darebee.com
20 seconds each exercise | no rest between exercises

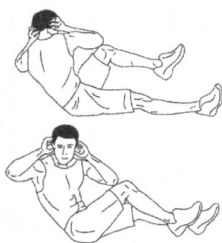

knee-to-elbows

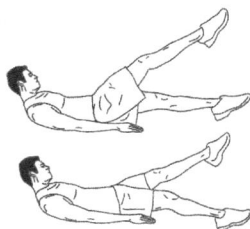

flutter kicks

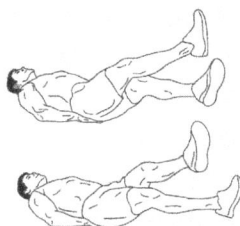

scissors

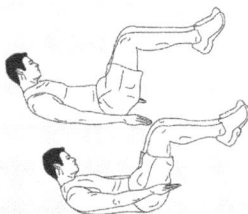

hundreds

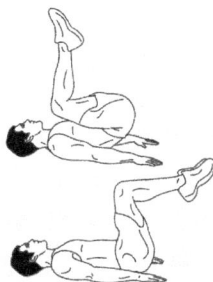

reverse crunches

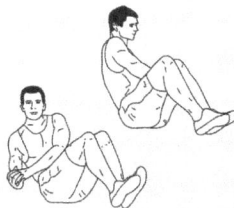

sitting twists

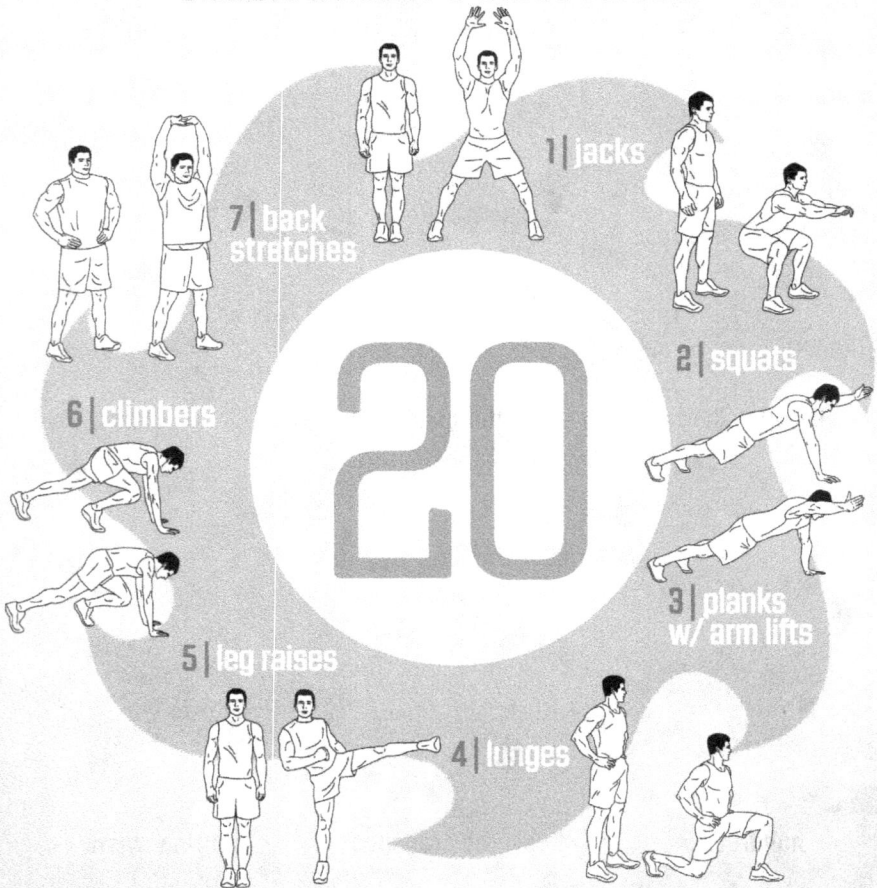

RISE & SHINE

DAREBEE WORKOUT © darebee.com

20

1 | jacks
2 | squats
3 | planks w/ arm lifts
4 | lunges
5 | leg raises
6 | climbers
7 | back stretches

THE GOLDEN OUTCOMES

The goals we seek acquire real meaning when we connect what we hold in our head with what we feel in our body. Without emotion no action is sustainable.

The traditional Vulcan goodbye in *Star Trek* is: "Live long and prosper". It's a brilliant wish to exchange with anyone you care for and one that's founded on the incontrovertible knowledge that time is against us. It robs us of strength and capacity because, over time we degrade.

If, indeed, we could live a long and healthy life then without a doubt we would succeed at pretty much anything we put our minds to. Yet, the majority of us will fail at this task. Some may live long but will fail to enjoy good health and will end up struggling to stay alive as long as possible through medication.

Others may enjoy good health but have a relatively short life.

The magic is when the two overlap so that we get to enjoy both a long and healthy life. As always, when this happens it is not by accident.

Statistically, genetics plays a part in this. But statistically, again, genetics plays a part in everything. There are so many complexities, variations, combinations and mutations in the human genome that in the mass of humanity on this planet there will always be some people who will enjoy good health and a long life without trying, they will not put on weight despite neglecting their nutrition and they will be relatively strong without engaging in a structured exercise program.

If you are one of these lucky genetic lottery winners, congratulations, You now have a headstart on the rest of us. Just because genetics has not handed us an instant win however doesn't mean there is nothing the rest of us can do.

The branch of biology called epigenetics studies the way our environment and our actions change the way our body reads the genes we do have and switches on or off specific traits from those genes to make changes that are beneficial to us. These beneficial changes happen when we engage in actions that specifically seek to help us attain the outcomes we would expect if we had been luckier in our genetic material and already had a guaranteed long and healthy life.

What this means is that provided we are willing to engage in intentional, structured activities and behavior that is designed to help us attain a long and healthy life, there is no reason for us to get ill and die before we are truly supposed to.

It sounds simple, I know. It isn't. And to understand why it isn't let's consider its exact opposite: dying. Fair warning, this chapter will sound a little grim, but it has to if we are to understand what we have to do so as not die young.

Death Is A Weird Idea

I am going to start by telling you a truth you already know: you are going to die. So am I. We are all going to die. I know that reading this makes you feel uncomfortable. It made me feel uncomfortable writing it. And yet this is the only certainty in our life.

Death is a weird idea because we spend so much of our time, energy and inner resources trying to predict the next possible moment as accurately as possible so that we reduce the uncertainty that surrounds it and increase our chances of survival and yet when faced with the one single thing we can be absolutely certain about, our brain shies away from thinking about it.

In 2019, just as the COVID-19 pandemic was starting to spread, a group of researchers from the Gonda Brain Research Center of the Bar Ilan University in Israel and the Lyon Neuroscience Research Center of the Lyon University in France were busy testing the responses of volunteers of different ages, sexes and socioeconomic background to the idea of their own mortality.

What they discovered is that our brain has a death-denying mechanism that kicks into gear each time we get an intimation that we might die. It's not that logically we don't know it will happen. As I said just a little earlier this is the one thing we can all agree on, but we feel uncomfortable even contemplating it and our brain places it in the cabinet where it holds things that happen to other people.

Crazy as it may sound, we all understand death exists but we all also feel that it won't happen to us any time soon so we can safely not worry about it.

No one yet knows how that mechanism works in our brain. Researchers can see the parts of the brain that are triggered and they can measure the outcome of that triggering by quantifying the response of the subjects to ideas and associations that intimate that they too can die.

The reason we are examining this now, here, is because this mechanism inadvertently also makes us neglect our health, ignore our mental well-being and fail to plan our diet.

Like so many other mechanisms we have examined here that undermine our efforts to get physically and mentally strong and healthy this too, in the ancient past served a crucial purpose and it may still do.

By acknowledging the inescapable reality of our death we might be tempted to question the point of our own existence. Because there is no real answer to that we could become distracted and maybe even depressed and we know that distraction alone, never mind depression, would immediately make us less efficient. It would affect our capacity to function on a day-to-day basis and it is more than likely that it could also negatively impact our immune system.

Is there a middle ground? Can we learn to balance the certainty of our death with the plan to live a full, healthy, fruitful and intentional life? The answer to that question has already been given. In his 1998 book, *The Greatest Generation* American author and NBC News anchor, Tom Brokaw, used the term "the Greatest Generation" to recognize the fact that the post-war era gave us "a generation of towering achievement and modest demeanor, a legacy of their formative years when they were participants in and witness to sacrifices of the highest order.... This is the greatest generation any society has produced."

These were people who in America and around the world had experienced a great depression that robbed countless millions of the means to make a living. Those who survived it were then subjected to the horrors of the second World War and, in its aftermath, the Vietnam War and, in America, the Watergate Scandal.

The certainty of death and the imminence of dying was something people in that generation had to deal with first hand. The luxury of activating the death-denying mechanism in their heads was something that was denied to them by the reality of inescapable external events.

As a result the majority of people who lived through those times learned to live a full, healthy, fruitful and intentional life.

This supposition is backed by solid data. The 1970 British Cohort study is a research project set up to follow the lives of around 17,000 people born in England, Scotland and Wales in a single week of 1970.

The researchers discovered that the 1970 generation was more likely than those born in 1958 to report symptoms of poor mental health at age 42. Feeling depressed, anxious or irritable were common conditions with more men than women reporting a deterioration in mental health.

The findings of the study were published in the journal *Psychological Medicine* and they highlighted the fact that both men and women who had been born in 1970 appeared less able to regulate their emotions and manage their mental health than their peers who had been born just 12 years earlier.

Even worse, the rate of emotional disregulation and poor mental health in both men and women of the 1970 generation rises with each passing year, as they age.

In analyzing the results of their study the researchers noted that: "The rise in psychological distress is interesting given that the increase has occurred despite economic growth. However, the 1958 cohort are part of the 'Lucky Generation' of post-war baby boomers, who experienced high absolute levels of social mobility, and relatively low social inequality in their early lives, whereas the 1970 cohort are part of 'Generation X', who have experienced greater uncertainty and insecurity, and a more individualistic society."

What baby boomers experienced first hand were the results of actions that are not backed by an awareness of their effects. They were able to be as catalytic in the change they brought in society because they intimately understood what happens when no change is introduced and when social strata are allowed to become compartmentalized.

Note the differences here: baby boomers did not work harder than their children and their grandchildren. Their effectiveness in changing the world is not defined by their work ethic and we have studies to prove that or at least disprove the notion that they were the hardest working generation of our times. The reason for their effectiveness lies elsewhere.

That elsewhere has to, in part at least, reside in the awareness of their own mortality that came from their proximity to the war years and their direct contact with those who had lived through those war years and experienced, first-hand the hardship created by war and its aftermath.

Theoretical as this may sound it is backed up by what we know in terms of behavior and how that is formed through exposure to circumstances, people and experiences and the data we have which show that baby boomers are by far healthier than the generations that have come after them, despite the fact that those generations spend more time worrying about health than ever, have access to more information about health than ever and at least until the pre-Covid years, tended to live longer and longer with each generation thanks to advances in medicine.

It is a strong sense of awareness of mortality and life that has helped the baby boomer generation be as exceptional and consequential as it has been. Those born in the post-war years have lived full, healthy, fruitful lives and continue to redefine what old age looks like by exercising more in their third stage of life than Gen Z, for instance.

This brings me now to the second part of this chapter: healthspan.

I know you will agree with me that life is infinitely better when you don't have to worry about medical issues as you age. Living longer if it means suffering with poor general health and impaired mobility is not quite the gift it appears to be.

For life to feel exceptional and be amazing we need to have not just time, as in many years of life, but also good health during the years we live. Beyond good genetics and a little bit of luck is there something we can do to ensure that we live long and stay healthy enough to truly prosper?

As it turns out there is.

Healthspan

The subtext of the traditional Vulcan greeting with which I opened this chapter is that in order to prosper you need a long and healthy life. Vulcans in the Star Trek universe are such highly logical people that obviously they didn't think they needed to spell out the fact that a long life without good health is unlikely to lead to prosperity.

Healthspan is defined as the period of our lives during which we are free from any significantly debilitating disease.

There are three elements that contribute to our healthspan:

* Genetics
* Environment
* Lifestyle

There is a natural tendency to connect a long life with good health. Certainly people who live longer tend to be healthier. In the modern word however, our advanced medicine can keep us alive while we are in poor health for many years, through a variety of medical interventions.

We're at our happiest when we feel our best. And we feel our best when our body is strong and our brain is healthy. Everything in this book has in a step-by-step fashion helped you build your own blueprint for a long and healthy life.

Around the world there are specific geographical areas where the people who live there on average, live longer, healthier lives than the rest of the world. These are called "Blue Zones" and they include Sardinia, in Italy, the islands of Okinawa, in Japan, the island of Icaria, in Greece, Nicoya, in Costa Rica and Loma Linda in California, USA.

Each of these areas has a distinct culture, diet, lifestyle and arguably philosophy. What each has in common with the others however is the entire concept, or schema, of how they live. They're physically active every day, they have a varied diet that is low on red meat and high on whole plant-based foods, they drink little or no alcohol, they have a spiritual approach to life that gives them mental fortitude so they are resilient to life's challenges and they have strong communal ties and a good social network which helps them further control the stress they feel.

None of these characteristics, on its own, is exceptional. Yet, in their totality they safeguard the mental and physical health of the people who live there helping them remain younger than their biological age and keeping them healthier.

How do they do that exactly? How do the environmental factors that make all these things possible, and what are they? Again: physical activity, a varied diet low on red meat, plant-based foods, low-alcohol consumption, spirituality and a strong social network. How do these environmental factors contribute to something as tangible as a long and healthy life?

Genetics appears to make a 20% - 25% contribution to a long and healthy life. This leaves a whopping 75% within our influence. There are several key, overlapping and maybe, even, interacting mechanisms through which the genes we have, the environment, the food we eat and the physical activity we engage in influence each other; slow down the aging process of our cells and helps us stay free from major diseases. Epigenetics, the science that examines how our lifestyle choices, our environment and our level of physical activity affect the way our genes work, highlights the fact that many of these mechanisms are still poorly understood.

What we do know however points to a common underlying thread in all of them which is energy management in the body.

The concept is complex because the way the body manages energy, again, is not well understood and it is complicated to begin with. But the essence is simple: Our body needs a specific amount of energy to function each day. In that sense the food we eat is energy in (this is a gross oversimplification but it gives you the general picture) and the total of our activities in a twenty-four hour period, including sleep, is energy out.

Remember from earlier chapters that our body doesn't know that it can theoretically get an infinite amount of energy each day (and from a health point of view it is not a good idea that it should) so it changes to optimize the use it makes of the energy it has and the energy it gets.

Have we injured ourselves? We need energy to heal. Is there inflammation in our organs? We need energy to return them to a better functioning state. Do we lift weights? We need energy to build stronger muscles (and the energy-costly process of building muscles is itself an optimization strategy designed to reduce the amount of energy we use when we lift weights).

Anything that disturbs the way the body distributes energy throughout its systems is an issue. Disease, in its nuisance form like catching a cold, is a disruption in the way the body distributes its energy, which is why when we have a cold we can't usually train with the same intensity we do when we don't have one.

Disease, in one of its more serious forms like cancer or diabetes is a major disruption to the body's energy distribution system. A body that cannot distribute its energy as it needs to, malfunctions. It is easy, at this point, to think of energy used just when we move but that isn't what happens. The human body needs energy just to survive. Our 30 trillion plus cells need energy to carry out their daily function. If someone tied you up and left you on a spot for 24 hours, unable to move, you would still use up 1,500 plus calories just to stay alive.

If we imagine the body to be a perfectly formed organic and highly adaptive machine its long-term, malfunction-free function depends on its supply of energy remaining steady. Never too much and never too little and certainly no disruptions.

Now imagine what happens if we glut this machine with energy or we go the other way and starve it of energy or we disrupt the way energy flows through its vast network? This is exactly the kind of disruption that happens to our body when we overeat (or indulge in easy-energy foods like processed foods and sweets that are high in sugar), when we diet and when we become ill or when out internal tissues suffer from chronic inflammation.

Because physical activity is a means of managing energy in the body what we see happening in Blue Zone areas is the creation of an environment that makes varied physical activity a daily constant, transforms diet into something that provides energy that is not immediately available so it never floods our system and a communal setting that makes social connections easy.

Blue Zones across the world are usually small communities of just a few thousand people. This makes them easier to homogenize by way of social behavior and harder to disrupt by way of the behavior of a single individual or a small group of individuals. The setting they are in is embedded in nature. Those who live in them are exposed to the natural world on a daily basis whether they want to or not.

Most of us live in cities or areas that are larger than that as a result we have a lot less control over our environment and we are more likely to encounter unexpected events, have to deal with unforeseen problems and need to make decisions and choices that we cannot plan for beforehand. In addition, our surrounding environment is highly artificial. Man-made constructs surround us and we often work and live at a pace that defies the natural daylight hours and divorces us from the natural world.

The degree of disorganization we experience in modern life and its frenetic pace absorbs time and energy to navigate. This time and energy is then taken away from the time and energy we could devote to ourselves so that we too can experience the way of life and the benefits of those who live in Blue Zone parts of the world.

All of this helps us identify the real culprit behind much of what we experience that affects how we feel, what we do and how we end up.

From Sense To Health

Throughout this book, time and again, we've seen two things: That the body and mind are an indivisible and intertwined whole. What happens to one affects the other. And that the body's energy management system when balanced, is key to good health and a long, illness-free life. Key to this energy balancing act that's called homeostasis, are the brain's internal states that, for lack of a better popular description, we shall call them internal emotional predisposition or mood.

It feels like nothing less than a miracle to think that the moods we experience have the ability to affect our homeostasis and depending on the direction our moods point to, damage or help our health.

Japan, with almost a third of its population in the over 65 range, has the world's largest percentage of older people worldwide. To better manage the health of this segment of its population the country has made the practice of Shinrin-yoku or forest bathing, such a vital part of preventative healthcare that it's actually prescribed by doctors.

What the research shows is that forest bathing significantly contributes to a reduction in stress. Because chronic stress increases blood pressure and suppresses the body's immune response which leads to many other different diseases a reduction in that alone helps increase quality of life. But forest bathing also affects quality of sleep, our ability to focus and mood.

Kathy Willis, professor of biodiversity at the University of Oxford and author of *Good Nature: The New Science of How Nature Improves Our Health* writes in her book about studies carried out on patients in hospital beds who have a garden view out of their window which show that they experience less reported pain and recover faster than patients who have a conventional street view.

The body of additional scientific evidence that supports this has become so compelling that the Macarena University Hospital in Seville, Spain and the Derriford Hospital in Plymouth, United Kingdom are in the process of creating specific, stunning outdoor spaces for patients admitted to their Intensive Care Unit to help them recover faster.

What all this shows is that the environment we choose to expose our self to provides our body with a constant barrage of sensory information that our brain processes. This, in turn, becomes our perception of the world and how we feel in it. Our emotional state is expressed in complex neurochemical cocktails that affects our neurobiology.

We can use the sensory input we receive to help reset our health by re-balancing the internal states of our brain and body.

There are two competing theories on why we are made this way. The first one is called Biophilia and it was popularized by American entomologist and biologist, Edward O. Wilson in his 1984 book, by the same name. Wilson suggests that we evolved to live in nature and its presence, for us, is an integral part of who we are. When we live in artificial environments for a long time we suffer as a result and require exposure to nature to help us find our inner balanced state, again.

The other one is called Attention Restoration Theory and it was proposed, in the 1989 book called *The Experience of Nature*, by environmental psychologists Rachel and Stephen Kaplan. It argues that our ability to concentrate improves when we are exposed to natural environments because the exposure helps the brain restore the limited cognitive resources it uses to carry out its many tasks. This restorative action, essentially resets the brain's homeostatic thermostat, reduces stress and positively affects the body.

There are dozens of detailed studies supporting both theories so their inclusion here is purely of academic interest. What we really need to know is that exposure to nature, whether real or virtual, works to restore our inner balance and help us feel more in control of our life.

Since it is the relative chaotic experience of modern life with its constant demands on our attention, that gives us the sense that we lack control over our life that generates these inner imbalances and it is stress that makes us ill, we can work backwards. By starting from where we want to end up in life, how we want to be and how we want to feel we can put in place the steps, choices and actions required to make it happen.

Plan Your Healthspan

Like most desirable outcomes that have a high value in our life we need to plan for this one too.

To help you plan your health better carry out this exercise, you will most probably need a few sheets of paper and a pen or, if you're digital, a tablet or phone with a note-taking app: Imagine yourself at age 60 or age 70. This is an age at which you would normally be described as being in your "advanced years". Now write down a list of things you would normally associate with that age. It will most probably include things like wrinkles, white hair (or no hair), some aches and pains and some physical malady that will almost certainly affect your mobility. Describe in as much detail as you can the physical fitness you think you will have at that imagined older stage of your life. Put in details like how fast do you think you'd be able to run, how high could you jump, how many squats could you do and how many push-ups? Add more details based on your direct experience or your direct understanding of exercise.

Now imagine what would that list look like if you were to subtract 20 years from that age. How would the things you've written change? Make those changes so you now have two lists you can compare.

The new list you created for a younger you is your target list for the older you.

Think, what steps can you take right now to make that happen? List them all. That is your healthspan plan.

Whatever it is, and it will be different for every person, it is still founded on three key principles.

- Energy
- Control of stress
- Control of environment

Implicit in this is the understanding that try as we might we shall all, still, have to face factors we cannot control. This makes it all the more important to have control over those factors we can control.

Because information first travels from the body to the brain, by modulating what we experience to make us feel good we create the emotional margin necessary to manage our emotional responses to the unpredictable events we do not control.

Essentially we unburden the brain from the energy load that comes with stress so that when something stressful does happen we have the capacity to deal with it without feeling that the sky is falling.

That is what Blue Zone environments do for those who live in them. That is how they manage to live long, healthy lives even though they do not have an abundance of resources or an absence of stress from their life.

This is something you can create for yourself, too.

Take Action

Problem: Old age, ill-health and physical weakness is something that creeps up on us, incrementally, over time. Because of its slow, progressive nature we are both unwilling and incapable of noticing unless we are actually paying attention and are active architects of our own life trajectory.

Solution: The key to achieving a long, healthy and fulfilling life lies in the ability to articulate how long, healthy and fulfilling the life we want should be. It is only by paying attention to what is happening to us, physically and mentally, each day that we can begin to take control over our mind and our body.

Action Plan

Unless you are intentional in how you live you are unlikely to be able to exercise control over your life. Intentionality is created through self-awareness of our actions and accountability of their effect. Small things like planning your day and sticking to your plan, decluttering your office and your home, keeping your possessions, like your car, clean, have an outsized impact on how we feel and, subsequently, how we act.

If you get into the habit of identifying the details in your life that soak up your energy and hold you back, you get into the habit of solving problems that stop you from being your best, performing your best and becoming your best.

Start by making a list of small, practical changes you can make in your life that will make your everyday reality easier.

It could be, as a suggestion, pre-planning all your lunches so that your nutrition is always on point. Or, you could simplify the color coding of your wardrobe so you make it easier to pick your outfits every morning.

You could, if your budget allows it, automate some tasks around the house:

from creating routines on a smart home hub of when lights should go on and and off and when background heating or cooling should turn on to getting an AI-assisted floor cleaning robot like Roborock or Roomba or any of the other quality brands that package smart processors into their hardware. This would free up time you spend doing menial tasks without sacrificing the cleanliness of your home.

Expand this approach and thinking to other aspects of your work and home life. For example, a friend who lives on his own, worked out that it was cheaper for him to use disposable paper plates and a paper cup for dinner each night than have dishes piling up or having to worry about doing the dishes afterwards and he did the same thing when he invited me and a few other friends over for a casual get-together, one evening.

Aim, wherever you can and always within your means, to feel freer in how you live by shedding some of the menial, draining tasks of your everyday life.

We live longer and become healthier through the physical adaptations we trigger in our body as a response to the actions we undertake. The following eight DAREBEE workouts have been specifically designed and field-tested to push your body a little so that the adaptation response is triggered a little more easily. They include a good mix of aerobic, resistance, mobility and high intensity, interval training (HIIT) workouts, for better all-round results.

THE
CENTENARIAN

DAREBEE WORKOUT © darebee.com

LEVEL I 3 sets **LEVEL II** 5 sets **LEVEL III** 7 sets **REST** up to 2 minutes

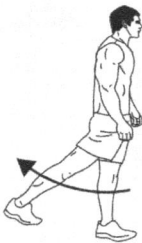

20 straight back leg swings **10** hip rotations **20** alternating chest expansions

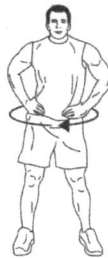

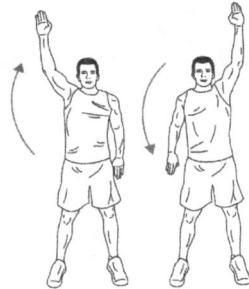

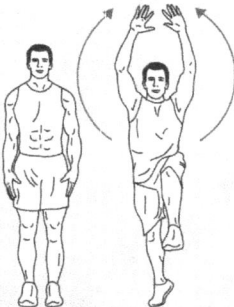

20 march jacks **20** side jacks

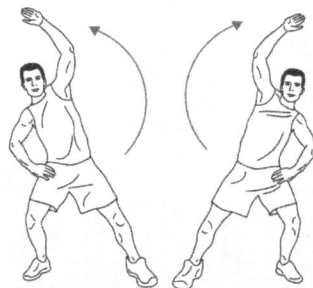

POWER PUMP

DAREBEE WORKOUT © darebee.com

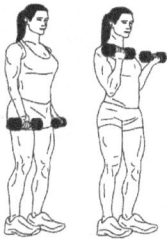

12 bicep curls x **5 sets**
60sec rest between sets

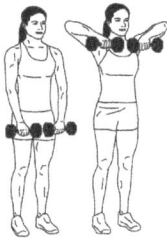

8 upright rows x **5 sets**
60sec rest between sets

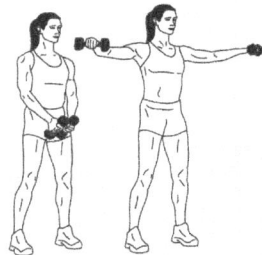

8 lateral raises x **5 sets**
60sec rest between sets

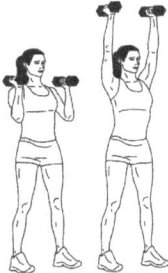

8 shoulder press x **5 sets**
60sec rest between sets

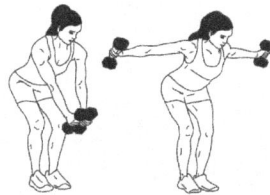

8 bent over raises x **5 sets**
60sec rest between sets

ANTI-AGING
MOBILITY

DAREBEE WORKOUT © darebee.com

LEVEL I 3 sets **LEVEL II** 4 sets **LEVEL III** 5 sets **REST** up to 2 minutes

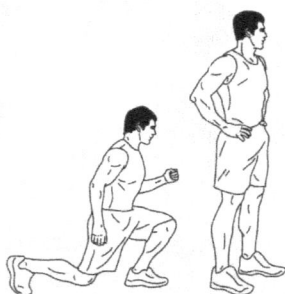

10 reverse lunges

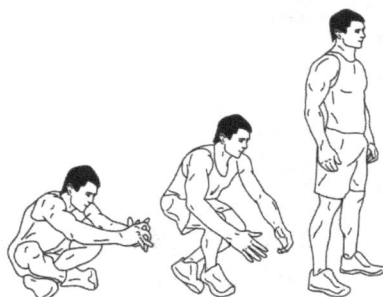

10 sit-to-stand

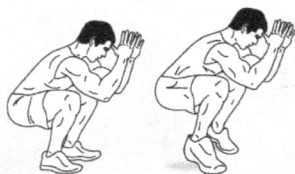

10 squat toe rolls

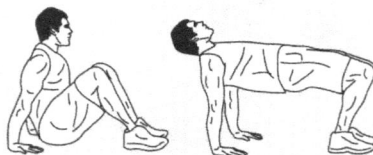

10 full bridges

CANNONBALL

DAREBEE **HIIT** WORKOUT © darebee.com

Level I 3 sets **Level II** 5 sets **Level III** 7 sets | 2 minutes rest

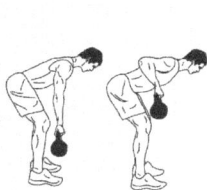

20sec bent over rows

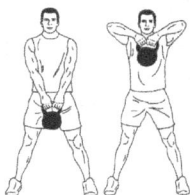

20sec upright rows

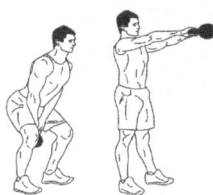

20sec swings

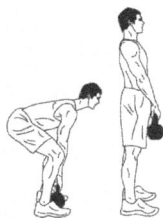

20sec deadlifts

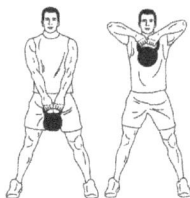

20sec upright rows

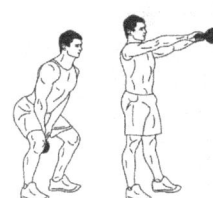

20sec swings

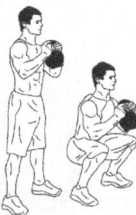

20sec squats

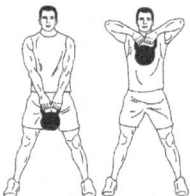

20sec upright rows

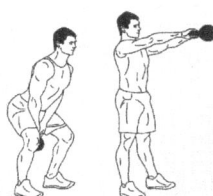

20sec swings

cardio MAX

DAREBEE WORKOUT © darebee.com

LEVEL I 3 sets **LEVEL II** 5 sets **LEVEL III** 7 sets **REST** up to 2 minutes

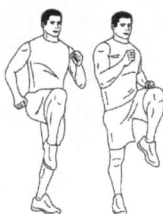

10 high knees

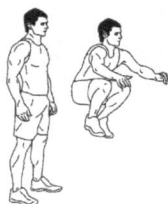

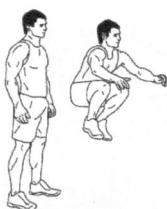

5 jump knee tucks

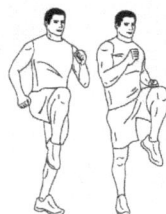

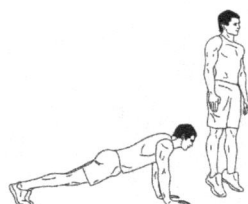

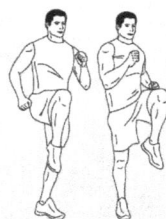

10 high knees

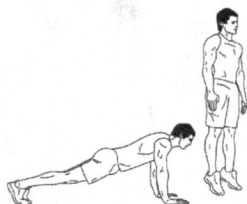

10 basic burpees

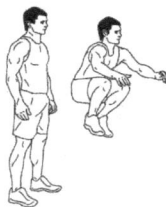

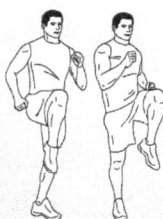

5 jump knee tucks

10 basic burpees

10 high knees

5 jump knee tucks

10 high knees

Cardio High

DAREBEE WORKOUT © darebee.com

LEVEL I 3 sets **LEVEL II** 5 sets **LEVEL III** 7 sets **REST** up to 2 minutes

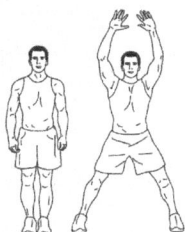

20 jumping jacks

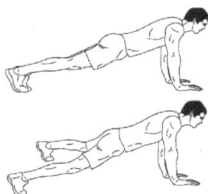

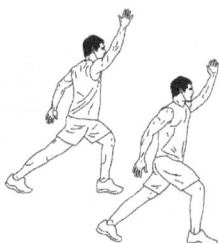

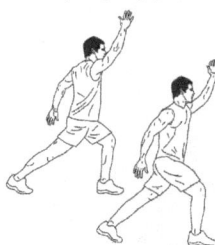

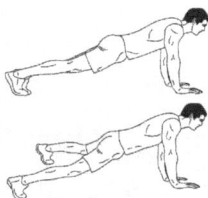

20 plank jacks

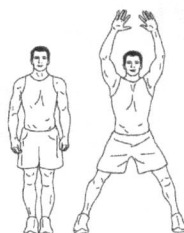

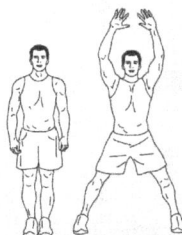

20 jumping jacks

20 split jacks

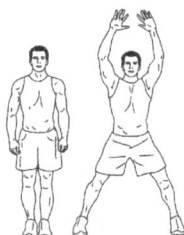

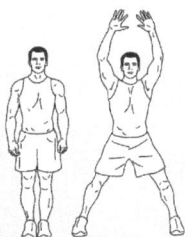

20 jumping jacks

20 split jacks

20 jumping jacks

20 plank jacks

20 jumping jacks

SIZE UP

DAREBEE WORKOUT © darebee.com

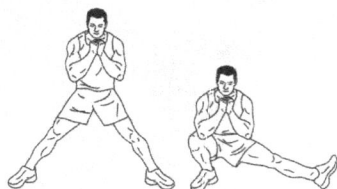

16 cossack squats
5 sets | 30sec rest

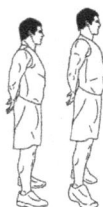

16 calf raises
5 sets | 30sec rest

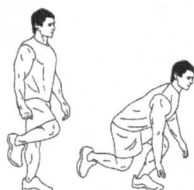

16 single leg squats
5 sets | 30sec rest

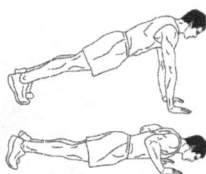

max push-ups
5 sets | 30sec rest

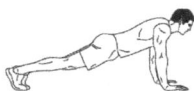

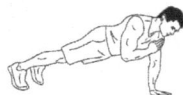

16 shoulder taps
5 sets | 30sec rest

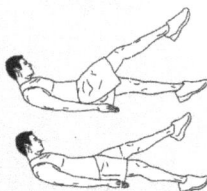

16 flutter kicks
5 sets | 30sec rest

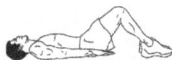

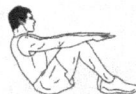

16 sit-ups
5 sets | 30sec rest

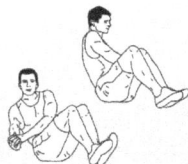

16 sitting twists
5 sets | 30sec rest

TURBOCHARGED

DAREBEE HIIT WORKOUT © darebee.com
Level I 3 sets **Level II** 5 sets **Level III** 7 sets | 2 minutes rest

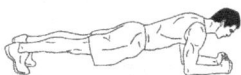

20sec elbow plank hold

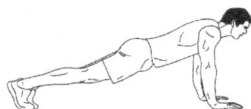

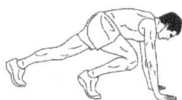

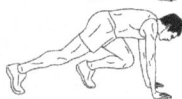

20sec plank hold

20sec climbers

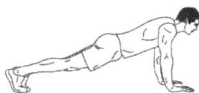

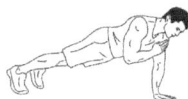

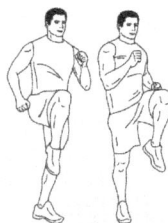

20sec shoulder taps

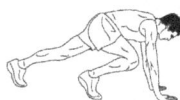

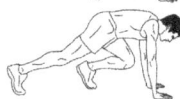

20sec climbers

20sec high knees (sprint!)

The four DAREBEE workouts that follow are not energy-intensive at all, but they all work the body/mind connection, help trigger adaptations that slow down the aging of the body and deliver dexterity gains that increase the overall sense of capability we have and our own sense of well-being.

GRIP
TRAINING

DAREBEE WORKOUT © darebee.com

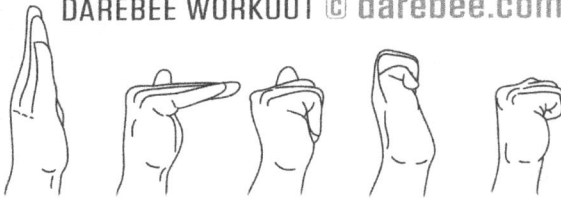

arrow - into - **table top** - into - **straight fist** - into - **claw** - into - **fist**
repeat 10 times in total

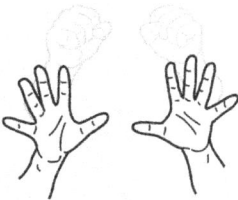

60sec clench / unclench **60sec** dumbbell hold #1 **60sec** dumbbell hold #2

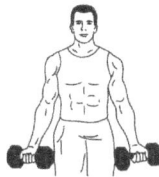

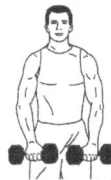

optional
but recommended

20 seconds deadhang
3 sets | 60 seconds rest

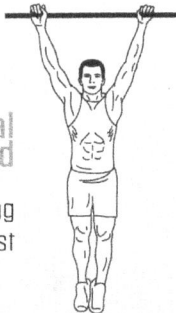

rainmaker

DAREBEE `OFFICE` WORKOUT © darebee.com

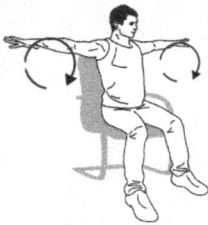

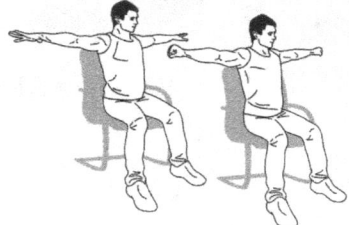

20 side circles   **10-count** hold   **20** side clenches

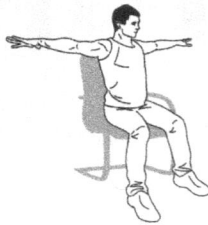

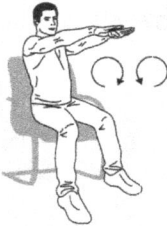

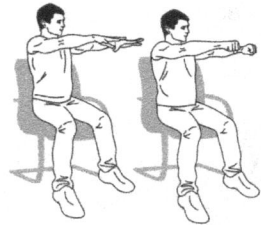

20 forward circles   **10-count** hold   **20** forward clenches

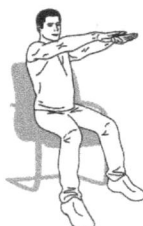

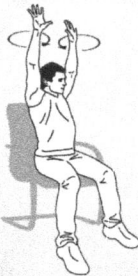

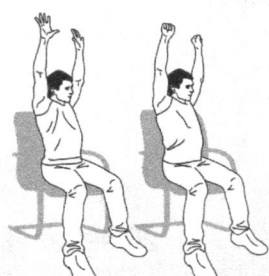

20 overhead circles   **10-count** hold   **20** overhead clenches

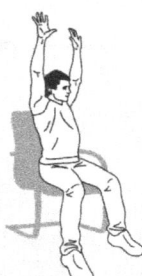

DEXTERITY

DAREBEE
WORKOUT
© darebee.com
LEVEL I 3 sets
LEVEL II 4 sets
LEVEL III 5 sets
REST up to 2 minutes

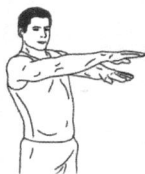

10 arm scissors

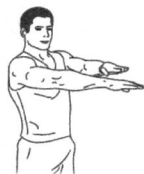

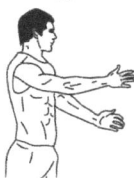

10 scissor chops

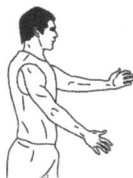

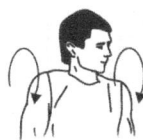

10 shoulder rotations

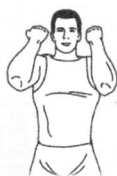

10 bicep extensions

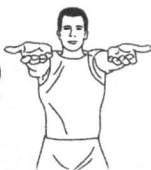

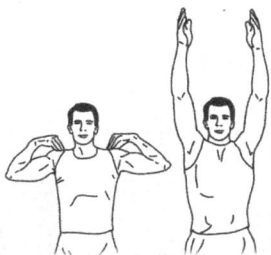

10 shoulder taps

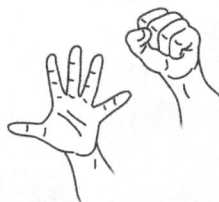

30 clench / unclench

Catch & Release

DAREBEE WORKOUT
© darebee.com

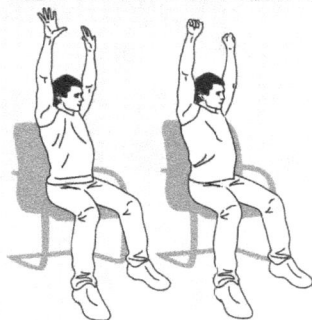

overhead clench
20

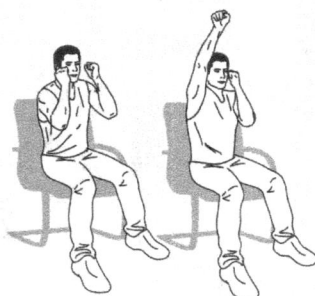

overhead punches
20

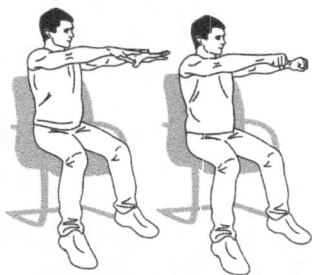

extended clench
20

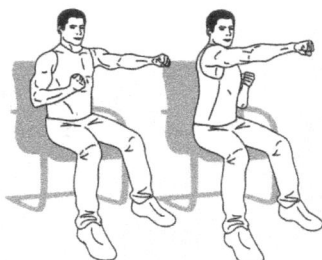

punches
20

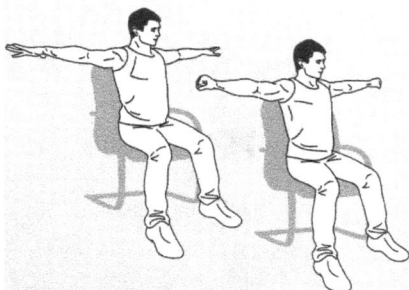

side extended clench
20

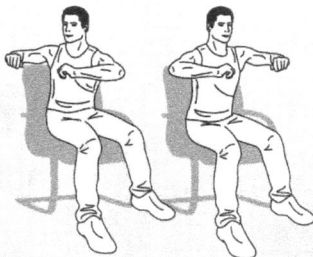

torso twists
20

THE OBSTACLES

The goals we pursue escape us when we fail to take full responsibility for the process that will help us achieve them.

We are strongly tempted to 'wing it' when it comes to fitness. We usually wrap fitness-related activities into 'fun' and anything fun, we feel should be spontaneous and unstructured. But everything that lacks structure, especially an activity, is haphazard and makes it difficult to measure its effectiveness. Fitness, in order to work best for us requires structure.

Logical as this may sound it stumbles upon the obvious obstacle called life. The mix of structured and unstructured, planned and unexpected challenges life throws at us exhausts us. As a result planning the structure of an activity that is supposed to be fun requires energy we don't usually feel we have. The mere thought that this too, now, has to be part of a disciplined approach to life, exhausts us before we even start to properly design anything that has to do with it.

What are we to do?

Obviously a rethinking or at the very least a reframing of our approach is required. Fitness and health are too important to be left to chance. Winging it, doing it when we can and when time allows or using hope as a strategy as in: we hope to get some time in the future, we hope to be able to do what we need in order to get fitter and feel healthier, are not a sound approach.

At the same time it is important to maintain the spontaneity and fun element of fitness and health. It is really important to shed the mental load we shoulder every time we think of things we "must do" or "should do".

Fitness, remember, is something that was inevitable for us in the past as part of the active lifestyle necessitated by our environment. We didn't plan it and we didn't structure it. If anything, and this is supported by ethnographic field studies of the few existing hunter-gatherer tribes left in the world, we sought to avoid it by resting as much as possible.

So it is our modern lifestyle that's basically causing the problem. We have no time machine to go back in time, nor would we really want to if we did. At the same time it is up to us to use that other weapon evolution has given us: intelligence, and work out a smart way to build up our health and improve our fitness.

I know what you're thinking: this sounds like extra work already. And life is already hectic. You're right, of course. The smart thing to do when facing an obstacle, and life places many obstacles that stops us from getting healthier and being fitter, is not to work harder to get over it but to work smarter and get around it or make it disappear altogether.

In order to do this we need to know what are the obstacles that are most likely to pop up as we try to stay strong and healthy for life. Once we know them we shall examine what we can do to make them disappear or successfully bypass them. Broadly speaking the obstacles we face are going to fall into one of two categories: Structural (and practical), psychological (and conceptual).

Sometimes, if our luck is bad because we haven't yet saved enough kittens in this lifetime, we may experience a combination of obstacles that come from both these categories. These are the hardest ones to solve or bypass for reasons that will become abundantly clear further into the chapter. But let's look at the easier ones first.

The Mind Trap

The most powerful organ we have in our body is our brain. What we think and feel about exercise and our health helps us determine what we are prepared to do to safeguard it. When we are truly focused on what we want to achieve and we are in what we call a "dialed-in" state, nothing can stop us from achieving it.

Unfortunately, at the same time, the brain which is our greatest strength, turns out to be our greatest weakness. It often twists us into knots of perception and expectations. I will give you an example: you're training at the gym. You trained hard the day before at home. Really hard. You pushed yourself to the limit doing body weight exercises to help you develop power and speed. You now go to the gym to work on upper body strength using equipment you don't have at home.

You have specific things in mind to do that take into account the fact that you have not fully recovered from the session you did the day before so, quite sensibly, you want to build on what you did at home.

However, when you get to the gym it is full of lifter types. Wherever you look there is someone granting and moving some unreal amount of weight. What do you do?

Well, if you're truly dialed-in you will get on and do your thing, but this is not usually what happens. What usually happens, and this is backed by social psychology studies, is that our perception of our body and its fitness and its capability is guided by the social group norms we are exposed to.

Within minutes of entering that lifter's gym and starting your session you will find yourself grunting and grimacing as you push your body beyond that day's safe levels of performance as you try to match what you see around you.

We fear being judged and we are afraid of sticking out or not fitting in and this often trips us up when it comes to intensely personal and arguably selfish goals such as getting fitter and feeling stronger. This mental jury of our peers that has us under a spotlight the moment we enter a public space is guided by a fierce judge that will brook no weakness from us.

Successfully dealing with it is a matter of reaffirming what is important to us and then framing that in a context that acknowledges the value of what we do and does not reject the society we live in. For instance we can acknowledge that fitness is a journey, not a destination. There is never an 'arrival'. We are all therefore at different places of our own personal fitness journey. We each train for what we want to achieve in that moment and to allow ourselves to be swayed by the fear of being judged by others is to be untrue to our self which means we shall be forced to abandon our fitness journey.

This simple reframing allows us to deal with the perception of peer pressure and social judgment on terms that do not impact our self image and do not affect our well-being.

Since we're talking about well-being it's useful to discuss injuries because, when they happen, they're the biggest obstacle we have to overcome. Strictly speaking an injury happens when a certain part of our musculature is exposed to more physical stress than it can tolerate. So we basically exceed our performance limit. When you're thinking about this keep in mind that the physical limits we have will vary from one day to the next. We're really not machines with fixed performance parameters.

Our body is wired to help us survive which means it is also wired to avoid injury. So, when we get injured it's because we ignored all the warnings the body gave to us.

We ignore the warning signs of injury because we feel our body is betraying us and we often and stupidly try to "train through" whatever pain signals it is sending us. There are countless examples in research literature: Runners running with bad knees. Lifters lifting with pulled ligaments and tendons. Boxers and martial artists pushing through the pain of muscles that have suffered mechanical damage due to tension and need rehabilitation and rest.

When someone does a sport for a living we can perhaps understand a little better their reticence to acknowledge that their body is failing them. When, however, we exercise for health and recreation it makes a lot less sense.

It's a fact that if we applied three basic, reasonable steps every time we felt a warning signal from our body we would never, ever get injured during exercise. What are those three steps?

- Identify what the pain (signal) is.
- Understand what caused it or what might have caused it.
- Put in place specific actions that will fix it.

This, of course, presupposes two other things:

- We must learn to listen to our body. And by 'listen' I mean understand it. Not as a biomechanical instrument that's there for us to use at will but as a complex construct that has emotions, feelings and thoughts which influence the way it behaves and the way it operates.
- We must be kind to it. No "training through pain" like some sort of deranged task-master when the pain we experience is the result of some underlying injury or it is caused by a muscle or tendon that are being pushed to their performance limit.

Both listening to our body and being kind to our self are different sides of the same skill. Our body is the place where we live. If we cannot familiarize ourselves with it so that we know its moods and quirks and signals then we shall never be able to guide it like a coach. And guiding it like a kind, knowledgeable and determined coach is what we need to be able to do.

Realistically we need all that in order to have the sense of control necessary to mitigate runaway anxiety and out-of-control stress from harming our health and destroying our fitness. But we also have to be able to listen to our body and be kind to ourselves so that internally our system can achieve the homeostasis necessary to reduce its energetic load.

Remember it is homeostasis that allows us to feel at peace in the world. It is homeostasis that resets us and allows us to survive everything that unbalances our system. It is homeostasis that allows us to feel happy not just inside our own skin but just happy in general.

To achieve the homeostasis we need for our own internal balance, we must have a plan on how to deal with the obstacles that cross our path.

Structural Obstacles

Structural obstacles that block our path to lifelong fitness and a happier life fall into two main categories:

- Physical
- Resource-driven

As the name implies physical obstacles are ones we experience at a personal level. They are obstacles we experience with our body and mind and stop us from engaging in exercise because of practical considerations that need to be overcome. Resource-driven problems usually come down to the lack of something. They are perceived obstacles because we think we cannot exercise because we don't have something we think we need.

Notice how I stress perceived and think. I do that because most structural problems we face that stop us from doing what is good for us but which requires some effort can be overcome with a little ingenuity and some planning.

This One Is Gonna Hurt

How many times have you heard the phrase "no pain-no gain" associated with physical exercise? While there is a very specific context with very specific goals that make this phrase make sense, every other time it shouldn't even be uttered let alone passed along like wisdom.

Exercise should not hurt and gains in fitness don't have to be paid for with pain. Exercise should be fun and if it is fun it becomes a consistent habit. It is consistency that provides gains in fitness not the pain we experience while exercising.

It needs to be said that the most obvious block to exercising and getting healthier is pain. Because we are hardwired to avoid pain if we come to associate exercise with it we are just setting ourselves up to fail. The avoidance we will feel inside our head each time we think about exercise is going to be so intense and persistent that we are unlikely to ever create a habit of exercising.

If we're experiencing pain because we are pushing the limits of what we can physically do we are also increasing the risk of injury.

Injury is a serious obstacle. If you get hurt exercising, depending on the severity of the injury any or all of these things in any combination you care to consider may happen:

- Your fitness journey will be derailed.
- Your mobility will suffer.
- Your confidence in your self will take a hit.
- You will become demoralized.
- You will give up fitness for a while.
- Your experience of the benefits of physical training will be tainted.

Injuries do happen when exercising. In non-competitive sports however they are the result of carelessness and the lack of awareness and I shall address both of these things now.

Carelessness in physical training is both spontaneous and cultivated and it has its roots in two emotions: guilt and hope. We become careless in the way we use our body when we feel guilty because we don't exercise enough and when we hope that by increasing the intensity of what we do we can get away with doing harder things in a shorter time.

A little exercise is always better than nothing but if you want to be injury free you will need to be your own coach who holds nothing but your own best interest at heart. World-class sports clubs and world-class athletes hire coaches not to motivate them (they're already highly motivated, that's how they got where they are in the first instance) nor to help them train (they're already pushing the limits of what they can do in every way they can) but to protect them and help them develop their physical fitness without incident.

That's what you really need to do for yourself now. Instead of listening to that inner voice that's guilting you for not doing enough and it's telling you to push harder, you need to be a kind, gentle, nurturing coach who will say: "Let's see what you can do without pushing it, let's test things gently, let's go slow but steady,"

Without exception injuries in physical exercise occur for two reasons:

- We push past our physical limit.
- We have ignored the warning signs of an underlying injury.

Injury is not feeling sore the day after hard exercise. It is not feeling bruised and having joints and muscles ache as you move a day or two after training. Injury is the structural breakdown of muscle, ligament or tendon or the fracture of bone because it has been pushed past its safe functional limits.

Injury happens when we push too hard without first having put in the time and work necessary to build up the required strength or when we ask muscles, tendons or ligaments to perform their best when they suffer from small problems: aches, pains and reduced function that are real warning signs that something is wrong.

In an ideal, but not unrealistic scenario, we can train all our life without ever getting injured. Here's how:

- Be aware of your body - learn what its signs tell you by listening to it instead of ignoring it.
- Train for consistency rather than intensity - you may want to test yourself from time to time but training every day (or as near every day as you can) will help you remain strong, healthy and injury free.
- Add active rest days to your weekly routine - Never aim to go flat out and break personal records every day you train. That's unrealistic. On days when you are low because you experience higher than usual stress at work or have to deal with the complexities of life, illness or lack of sleep, you must have a contingency plan that's realistic (i.e. do light stretching, go for a walk, do some meditation, get some static stretching in while watching a movie).

Freefall

Boxing has often been called "the loneliest sport in the world". Inside a ring a fighter is alone. He has to face physical exhaustion, pain, fear and uncertainty and overcome them, on his own. Despite this a boxer is not alone. He has coaches for strength, speed and technique. Sparring trainers and sparring mates. A nutritionist and, if the boxer is successful, a psychotherapist. It takes the knowledge, experience and talent of all these people to make a successful boxer and that is before we start to count aides and corner men.

We make the decision to get fitter and healthier alone. Is it any surprise then that we so often fail? Is it any surprise that when we feel low we abandon our healthy habits? Is it any surprise that our fitness journey instead of being one marked with an ever increasing number of milestones reached, is one of starts and stops and starts, again?

What is surprising and what should be encouraging is the number of people who do restart after they stop. The loneliest sport in the world, if it was a sport, would be the attempt of the average individual to change the trajectory of their life and decide to get fitter and healthier so that they enjoy more of what life has to offer on their terms.

The question here is why do we believe we can succeed on our own when so many professional athletes never do what they do, alone? Maybe because of what we see: we see the boxer in the ring, on his own. His team and their work are not visible to us. We see the runner or the cyclist or the tennis player doing what they do alone and believe, erroneously as it turns out, that this is how they got where we can see them: on their own.

They didn't. Neither can we. They had help. So should we.

Sure you can, we all can, get very obstinate and angry and get down and say to ourselves: "This is it. I am going to get fit this year." Many of us do that at the start of each year and we have already seen the statistics for the failure rate of New Year Resolutions for fitness.

It's never that we don't want to. Nor is it that we cannot. It's all about the support we have when we are emotionally low, physically tired and psychologically spent. The need for someone to pick us up when we are down is real if we want to succeed in our fitness journey. Personally, I don't now have a nutritionist and a coach and a psychotherapist and I guess neither do the majority of you. So we need to fill the gap by being all those things to ourselves.

Is it a hard thing to do? Yes, for sure it is. Is it necessary? One hundred per cent. We all need to have that awareness of self where on a bad day, when the weather is bad, unexpected bills have come in, the day job was super-stressful and we have a cold, we have a contingency plan in place so that we can do some exercise instead of doing nothing and even if "doing nothing" on that particular day is our contingency plan because our stress levels are too high and our energy levels are too low (and you are the only one who can possibly judge that for your self), we can choose to do nothing without feeling guilty. Without feeling that we have failed. Without feeling that we're not worthy.

What stops us from going into freefall when we are low is the support network we have put in place and the ability we have developed to be our own cheerleader. That support network can take the form of family members who are rooting for us, or a friend we know we can talk to when we are in need. It might be an online forum where we have a connection with people we can trust and can vent without fear of judgment. It is up to you how you put your support network in place.

Know two things though: First, you will definitely need it. Second, if you have not got it set up, when things get bad and they inevitably will because life is messy, you will fail.

Plan To Succeed

It's true that if you fail to plan, then really you are planning to fail; even if that is not what you think you are doing. Planning is a skill and how good we get at it depends on many factors including our childhood home environment. At the same time planning is a way of prioritizing mental, emotional and physical resources.

If the day is not planned, if our fitness is not planned we are resigning ourselves to fate. Whether we manage to get a workout in or not on any given day will depend on factors we cannot control.

That is not a way to live life if you want your life to be a long and healthy one. At the same time I accept that sometimes planning in advance is going to be difficult, especially if the planning in question factors in variables like children and the potential disruptions that come with them, work-related crises or family problems.

I have a friend, let's call him Mark, who has a super-important job. He's really smart, responsible and knowledgeable about many subjects and he is aware that he needs to work on his fitness and his long-term health, particularly as he gets older. Fitness is his blindspot because, I suspect, he has an emotional reaction to his inaction.

In my discussions with him he came up with a whole lot of solutions: one was to get a gym membership. It's a start for sure but his erratic and admittedly heavy work schedule made this a non-starter from the beginning. Then he thought he'd work out on weekends by joining a cycling-club with another friend.

That was never going to work, as I pointed out, he was hanging the success of his quest for fitness and health on the uncertainty of the weather and the availability of another busy person. "Maybe I will go running now and then" he said. He does live near the sea but I already knew he's never been running and getting to run each day on your own when you've never done it was never going to work.

Finally, during our discussion, exasperated at my picking apart his fanciful plans for exercise, he said: "I will get an exercise bike."

Having access to an item of equipment that requires no other investment in effort to use is key to exercising whenever you can. Last time I saw him he'd lost some weight and was feeling a lot happier with himself and his life choices.

The point was that after some reflection (and my directness in pointing out the flaws in his plans) he was able to come up with the solution on his own:

- Make it easy to do.
- Make it accessible to get to.
- Make it automatic to complete.

The exercise bike is in his living room. He uses it while he watches Netflix on his TV. He often cycles for as little as 15 minutes after a meal because that's the only time he has but he does it every day.

If you plan your fitness you need to:

- Acknowledge the difficulties of your work and lifestyle.
- Find a way to remove most obstacles to working out.
- Accept that there will be days when even finding a whole hour to exercise is not an option.
- Have a contingency for the times when what you plan is not going to happen and you need an alternative.

Mark admitted to me that if he hadn't bought the exercise bike he wouldn't have had the time to exercise. Anything else would have required more commitment in time and effort from him that he just wouldn't have been able to make. Because he exercises regularly and enjoys the way it makes him feel he now finds that on days when work and life get messy and he cannot exercise he will still hop on his exercise bike, put the resistance up to the max and cycle like mad for two-three minutes.

That small contingency he has in place keeps him from feeling like he's stopped exercising on days when he can't. It stops him from feeling guilty and it actually helps him from a neurobiological point of view to maintain his fitness.

The body isn't aware of time constraints. When we exercise it undergoes a number of neurochemical changes that affect our internal organs.

These changes are largely the same whether we exercise for one minute or whether we are physically active for a full hour. Because these neurochemical changes are the same we can maintain the body's existing physical adaptations and maintain its ability to handle stress and deal with discomfort so that we remain emotionally regulated and mentally strong and resilient.

In the spirit of removing obstacles from the path of exercise in our planning you don't even, really, need any equipment. Have a pre-picked no-equipment workout you can do at home, or in the park or anywhere where you have a little bit of space. That way you don't even need to think about what you will do when you start to exercise.

For the days when you cannot find the time for that, have a back-up exercise plan. It might be as easy as ten push-ups or ten squats. Your back-up plan, your contingency, has to be easy to do, so it cannot be complex and it must make no demands on you by way of special clothes, special time of the day or a lot of space and it absolutely must require zero thinking.

Over time, this approach, will make a massive difference in how you feel, how you move and how you look.

Have A Destination

Fitness is a journey, not a destination. Nothing will ever be truer than this. Throughout our lives our body changes inside and out and our brain and central nervous system also undergo changes. We are never quite the same neurobiological being from one day to the next.

Fitness then is an on-going process. Our ability and what we do each day will evolve and adjust as we age and the horizon we reach for; shifts. Having said that it is also true that if you don't know where you're going any road will take you there.

This is where goals come in. If you don't have anything specific to aim for in the short-term you will be unable to measure your progress. When you can't measure your progress you're more likely to get discouraged, especially on days when you're already tired from work or other commitments and need to find the mental and emotional energy to exercise.

The thing to remember about goals is that they're like milestones. The moment they're reached we need to put fresh ones in place or embellish the ones we have already reached. Another friend of mine, for instance, set a goal to be able to do fifty push-ups in a row. He worked at it, in addition to everything else he did all year. It took him just over a year to actually get to it but when he did, he set himself a fresh goal of being able to do 100 push-ups in five consecutive lots of 20 with a 2-minute break in between.

Goals help keep you focused when everything else tends to distract you and exhaust you.

There is an art to setting goals and keeping them:

- Pick a fitness goal that means something to you, don't just go for something random.
- Set a fitness goal that is within reach of what you can do.
- Work at your goal in a consistent, structured way.
- Accept that you will have bad days.
- Celebrate your achievement when you reach it.

- Look for the next goal in line when you reach your current one.

One additional benefit of having a fitness goal is that it allows you to prioritize the attention and time you give to exercise. If your goal, for instance, is to run a half-marathon by a certain time, you're unlikely to go and do power-lifting with a friend just because he's into it and has invited you, nor are you likely to engage in any random exercise if it will not help you reach your personal fitness goal.

It's In Your Head

Conceptual obstacles in our fitness path are harder to address because we often don't see them and most times fail to really think about them. Yet, they undermine what we do and stop us from doing the exercise we hoped to do.

What's worse about them is that because they're mostly invisible they succeed in stopping us from getting fitter in ways that allow our brain, always adept at providing excuses that seem reasonable, to come up with excuses that seem perfectly legitimate. Excuses we can believe in as if they are truly what happened.

One such conceptual failure is the estimation bias.

Here's how this one works against us: if we're asked to determine the effort required to complete a specific task that requires mental or physical effort (or both) one of two things will happen, either we will underestimate the effort and difficulty of the task which means we're going to think that it is way easier than what it actually is, or we will overestimate its effort and difficulty which means we're going to think that it is way harder than it actually is.

What determines which side of the difficulty line our estimation of it falls on is how we feel at that particular moment in time. If, for instance, we're feeling fresh and relaxed and haven't got much on our mind we will use the "feel good" factor we are experiencing as the primary yardstick of our estimation.

Conversely, if we're feeling physically tired are mentally exhausted or are experiencing stress because of problems we are dealing with, we will use the sense of discomfort we are experiencing at that moment to estimate the level of difficulty of the task we are given and we will err on the side of it being "really difficult" even when it isn't.

The fact is that when we estimate the difficulty of a task and really we're talking about exercise here, although the concept holds true for any task we're asked to estimate, we are more likely to get it wrong than we are to get it right.

When it comes to exercise this is really important. If we have underestimated the difficulty and started off thinking something is going to be easy and, as we start to exercise, we begin to find it much harder than we thought it would be; our experience of it is going to be negative and we are unlikely to want to repeat it any time soon.

If, on the other hand, we overestimate the difficulty of the exercise we want to do, we are now facing a natural aversion to it because we are programmed to want to avoid activities that are likely to tire us out and exhaust our physical and mental resources so now we are faced with the additional difficulty of having to find extra energy, a stronger motivation if you like, to overcome the natural aversion we feel.

Other conceptual obstacles we will face come from social expectations. If, for example, we think that we should look a certain way when exercising (i.e. not sweaty, not gasping for breath, not heaving with effort) or if we think that our particular social group or society in general, expects us to breeze physical exercise then we also are unlikely to want to engage in something that we perceive to be hard and which makes us look bad.

Even positive behavior towards exercise, when unchecked, can be bad. Exercise, as we've already seen with my own personal example in chapter two, is a psychoactive mood modifier. Left unchecked it can become addictive. You may think that becoming addicted to exercise is a good thing, but addictive behavior by definition is harmful. It fails to recognize boundaries and it often delivers the opposite of the control we crave.

Addiction to exercise often leads to the same health issues with poor immune system, injuries and poor emotional regulation as having never exercised at all.

Conceptual obstacles are hard to overcome because they're so intimately tied into our sense of self, our own personal trauma and our own idea of how we want to be. Untangling them requires introspection, patience and above all a lot of kindness directed at our self.

By untangling them however not only do we remove some of the most persistent obstacles to our fitness we also take some real steps towards real personal growth.

Take Action

Problem: The things that stop us from feeling strong and being healthy are the obstacles we place in our way. Identifying them correctly is key to solving them. Some of them are tangible and practical. Others are imagined but nonetheless feel very real.

Solution: Learn to identify the things that keep you back and begin to quantify them so you can deal with them better. The best way to do this is to write them down and then break down each one into its component parts. This is the best way to solve practical problems. Conceptual ones are harder to deal with because they feel very real while they may not be. Their solution or mitigation requires an awareness of what is going on inside us. To better deal with stress or fatigue, for instance, we need to be able to recognize the symptoms they create in us and then have in place a strategy for dealing with them. It can range from finding ways to take quick breaks to reset or clever breathing strategies employed to help us decompress and refocus.

Action Plan

Focus on solving one or two practical problems at a time. Tackling everything at once is the best way to fail. Place a timeline on when they need to be solved by and detail the practical actions you will undertake. If, for instance, you want to exercise every day but fail to because of the complexities of life, detail a practical strategy for making this happen. Perhaps a walk at lunchtime. Maybe an exercise snack that is put into effect every day, before showering or every night, before going to bed.

To solve a practical problem you need to:

- Name the problem.
- List the actions required to solve it.
- Set a timeline (if that is required) by which you will have solved it.
- Track your progress every day.

If the problem is conceptual your approach will be a little different:

- Name the problem.
- List the actions (or strategy) required to mitigate it or solve it completely.
- Set a timeline (if that is required) by which you will have solved it.
- Track your progress each time you encounter it.

The following eight field-tested DAREBEE workouts focus on control, recovery and resetting your inner balance. They are great on days when you are not operating at a peak but still want to workout and help your body and mind feel better. As always, for the workouts that use dumbbells use ones you can comfortably lift or, if you don't have dumbbells; use a safe substitute weight instead.

24

DAREBEE WORKOUT
© darebee.com

YOU HAVE 24HRS TO COMPLETE YOUR MISSION

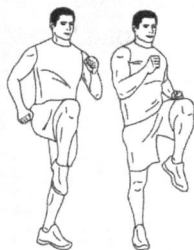

HIGH KNEES
120

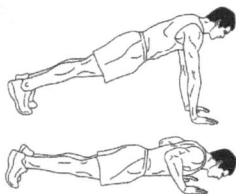

PUSH-UPS
60

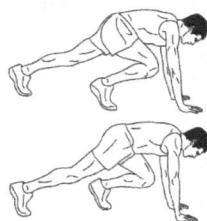

CLIMBERS
120

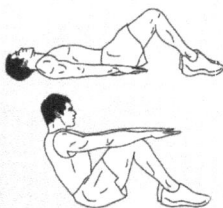

SIT-UPS
60

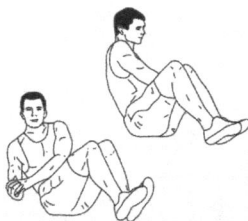

SITTING TWISTS
120

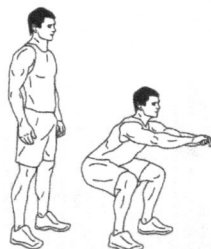

SQUATS
120

THIS IS MY
DAY OFF

DAREBEE WORKOUT © darebee.com

LEVEL I 3 sets **LEVEL II** 4 sets **LEVEL III** 5 sets **REST** up to 2 minutes

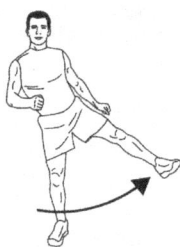

40 side leg raises

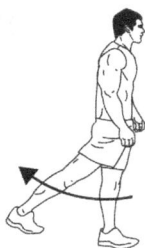

40 back leg raises

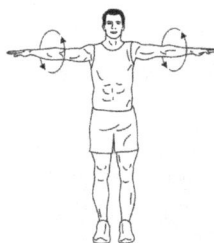

40 arm circles

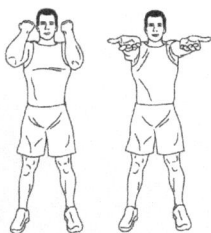

40 bicep extensions

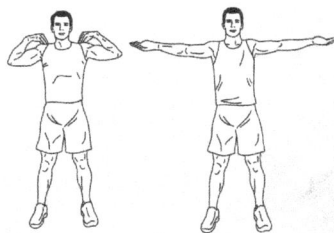

40 side shoulder taps

REST & REPAIR

DAREBEE WORKOUT © darebee.com

LEVEL I 3 sets **LEVEL II** 4 sets **LEVEL III** 5 sets **REST** up to 2 minutes

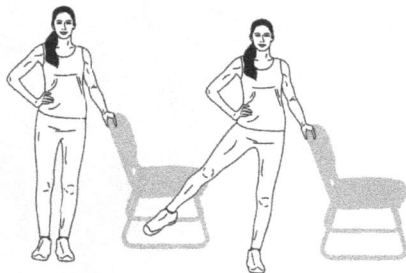

20 side leg raises

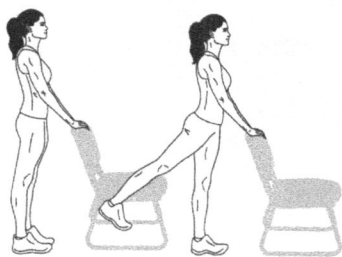

20 backward leg raises

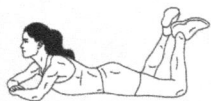

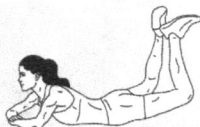

10 glute flex

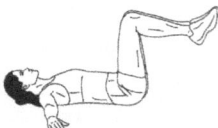

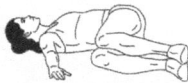

10 half wipers

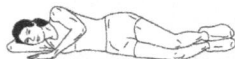

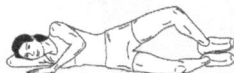

10 clamshells

ZOMBIES, WALK.

LEVEL I 3 sets **LEVEL II** 5 sets **LEVEL III** 7 sets **REST** up to 2 minutes

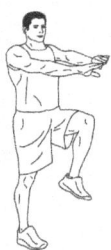

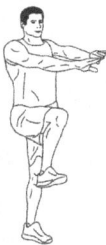

20 arms hold march

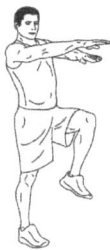

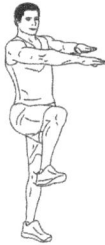

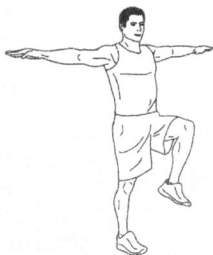

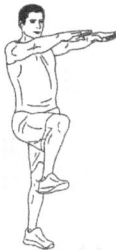

20 scissor march

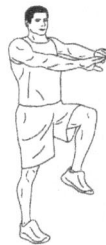

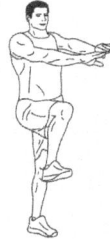

20 arms hold march

20 arm extensions march

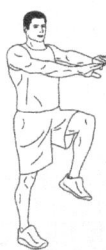

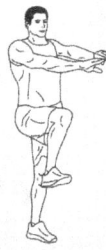

20 arms hold march

Seated Strength

DAREBEE WORKOUT
© darebee.com
LEVEL I 3 sets
LEVEL II 4 sets
LEVEL III 5 sets
REST up to 2 minutes

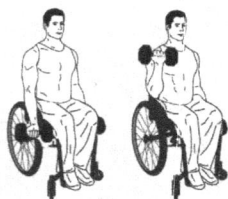

12 alt bicep curls

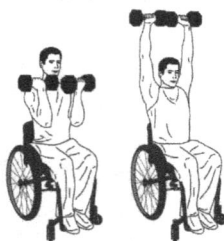

8 arnold press

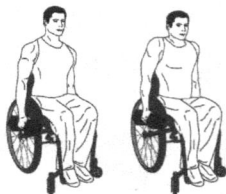

8 shrugs

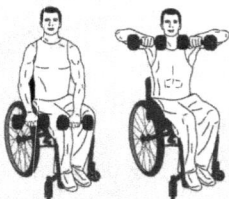

8 chest rows

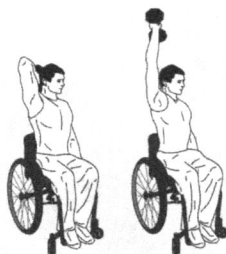

12 alt tricep extensions

ironclad abs

DAREBEE WORKOUT © darebee.com

LEVEL I 3 sets **LEVEL II** 4 sets **LEVEL III** 5 sets **REST** up to 2 minutes

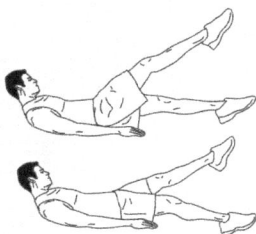

10 flutter kicks

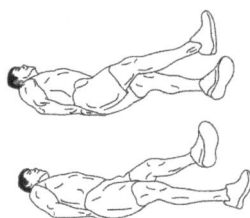

4 scissors

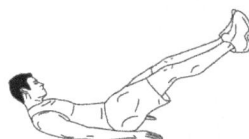

10-count hold

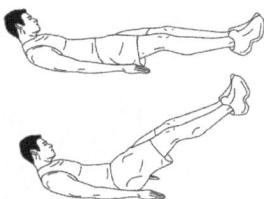

10 leg raises

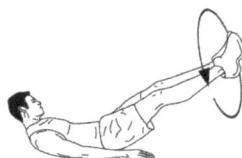

4 raised leg circles

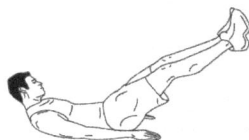

10-count hold

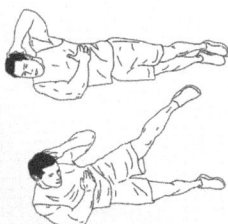

10 jackknives

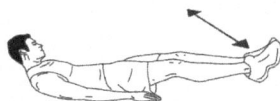

4 raised leg swings

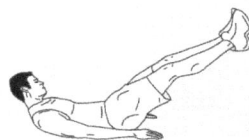

10-count hold

DAMSEL

DAREBEE WORKOUT © **darebee.com**

LEVEL I 3 sets **LEVEL II** 5 sets **LEVEL III** 7 sets **REST** up to 2 minutes

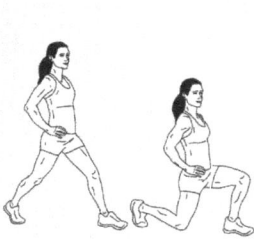

10 split lunges

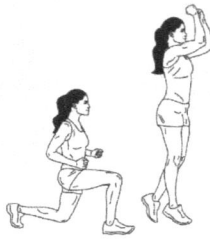

10 jumping lunges

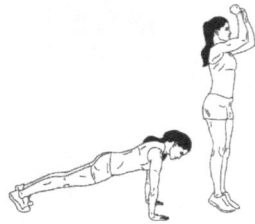

10 basic burpees

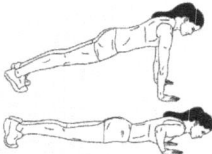

10 push-ups

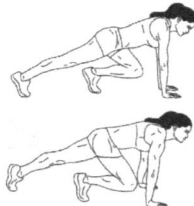

10 climbers

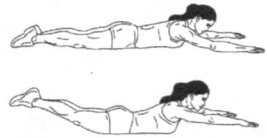

10 back extensions

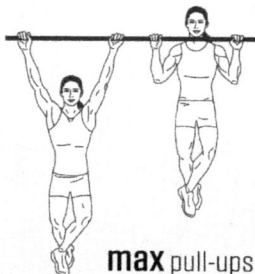

max pull-ups

lightning

DAREBEE WORKOUT © darebee.com

LEVEL I 3 sets **LEVEL II** 5 sets **LEVEL III** 7 sets **REST** up to 2 minutes

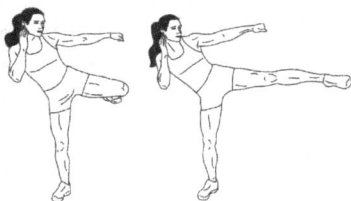

20 turning kicks

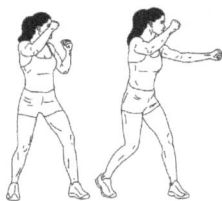

20 backfists

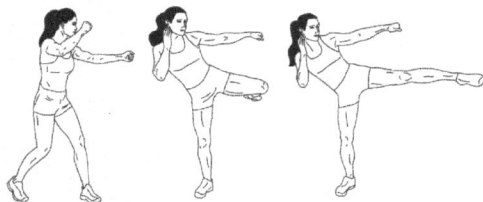

20combo backfist + turning kick

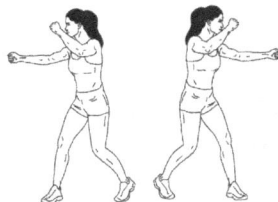

20 side-to-side backfists

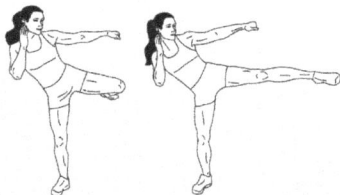

10 double turning kicks

The following four DAREBEE workouts that follow are your life-saver. Specifically designed to be quick and to the point, they are there for you to use on days when a longer workout is impossible either because you have no time or because you are low on energy.

DOPAMINE BOOST

DAREBEE WORKOUT © darebee.com

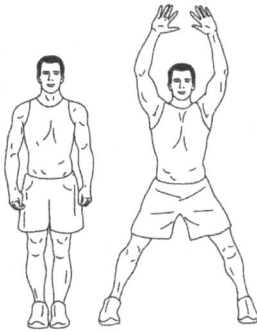

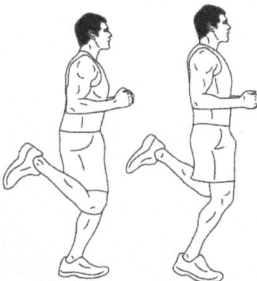

10 jumping jacks

10 butt kicks

10 jumping jacks

10 butt kicks

10 jumping jacks

10 butt kicks

10 jumping jacks

10 butt kicks

10 jumping jacks

10 butt kicks

5-MINUTE WALK

WORKOUT by DAREBEE © darebee.com

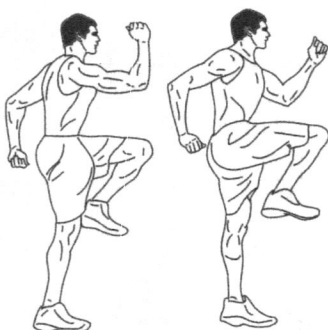

60sec march steps

15sec step jacks

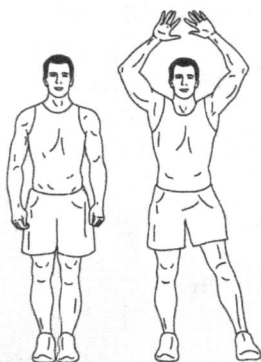

60sec march steps

15sec step jacks

60sec march steps

15sec step jacks

60sec march steps

15sec step jacks

RECOVERY WORKOUT

BY DAREBEE © darebee.com

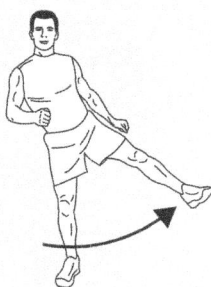

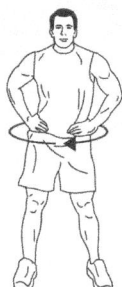

30 low side leg raises (right)
6 hip rotations (right)
30 low side leg raises (left)
6 hip rotations (left)

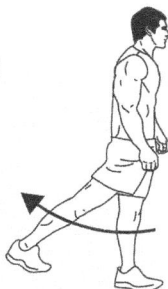

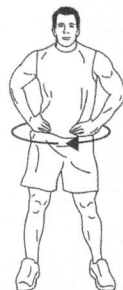

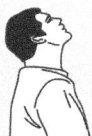

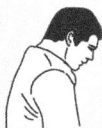

30 straight leg back swings (right leg)
6 hip rotations (right)
30 straight leg back swings (left leg)
6 hip rotations (left)

6 back and forth tilts   **6** side-to-side tilts   **6** neck rotations (3/3)

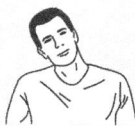

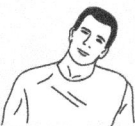

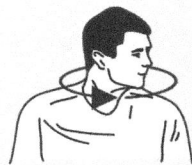

sore neck

DAREBEE WORKOUT © darebee.com

Repeat exercises #1-3 **6 times**.
Count to 10 while holding each stretch (for each side).

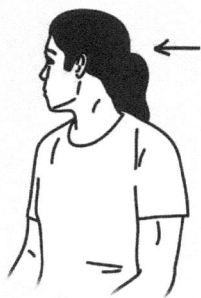

side-to-side turns

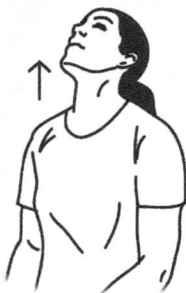

up & down nods

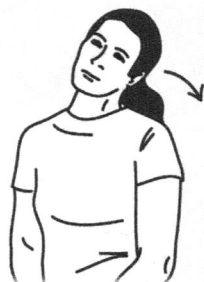

side-to-side tilts

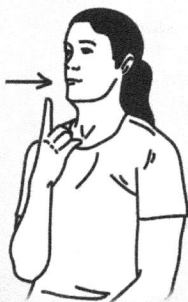

head back stretch

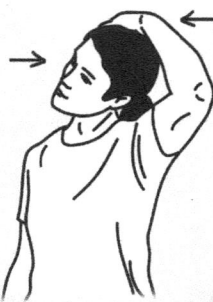

side stretch
(resistance)

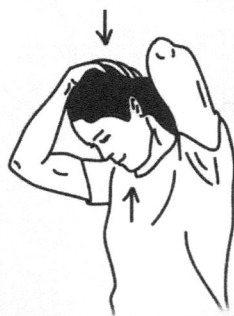

forward stretch
(resistance)

FINAL WORD

The only person truly responsible for your health and happiness is you. We tend to overlook this responsibility thinking "we're OK". This strategy works until it doesn't and we're no longer OK. But by then we are already feeling the impact of the neglect in our physical and mental health and looking for ways to fix it.

Fitness is important. It is also hard to do and extremely difficult to get right so that it is both sustaining and sustainable.

Our modern history of fitness is not long at all. Our knowledge of what works and what doesn't is expanding all the time and although we shed our misconceptions with difficulty, shed them we do.

If we want to have a long and healthy life we must make exercise an integral part of it. But we must also change how we feel about exercise, not just change what we do as exercise. How we do that is still left up to each individual. It's left up to you.

Ultimately, you are the one responsible for what you physically do and who you become as a result.

The workouts in this book have been hand-picked and field-tested by the global volunteer network of Darebee.com to give you a choice that fits in with most of your circumstances. But they are only the beginning. This book is only the beginning. In its totality this book opens the door into a new universe where you can begin your own, personal and amazing fitness journey to better health and greater happiness.

APPENDIX
ANTI-INFLAMMATORY FOODS

When it comes to using food to fight inflammation the John Hopkins School of Medicine and the British Heart Foundation both agree, the Mediterranean diet is highly potent when it comes to fighting inflammation. It is rich in antioxidants, trace elements, minerals and vitamins which have anti-inflammatory properties and it improves autophagy and Th cells imbalance which can lead to several forms of fibrosis.

Both research institutes however also point out that rather than trying t stick to a particular diet which can be hard due to access to some types of food and socioeconomic variables it is much better to try to have a varied diet that includes the following nutrients:

Omega-3: Fatty Acids. If you want to load up on omega-3s, fatty fish like salmon, herring, mackerel, sardines, tuna, striped bass, and anchovies are your best friends. You can get your fix by eating the fish itself or just take a fish oil supplement if that's more your speed.

Not into fish? No worries—there are plant-based options, too! Nuts, seeds, and even canola oil can help you get those omega-3s, plus a bonus dose of vitamin E (which also fights inflammation).

Vitamin C: Good ol' vitamin C (a.k.a. ascorbic acid) is a powerhouse antioxidant. It helps combat cell damage that can trigger inflammation.

You probably already know citrus fruits and juices are packed with vitamin C, but don't sleep on bell peppers—they've got a ton of it and come with fewer calories.

Polyphenols: Ever wonder why the Mediterranean diet gets so much love? A big reason is polyphenols—natural compounds found in colorful plant foods, whole grains, and olive oil that help fight inflammation.

And here's the best part: You can get your polyphenol fix from coffee, tea, and even dark chocolate. Yep, your daily caffeine habit just got a little healthier.

Gut-Healthy Foods: A happy gut = less inflammation. That's why it's important to keep your gut bacteria thriving with plenty of probiotics and prebiotics.

Just a heads-up: Not all fermented foods actually contain probiotics. Check the label to make sure it says "live active cultures." Yogurt and cottage cheese are usually safe bets, but always double-check the packaging.

RESEARCH

Chapter 1

1. Gallup. (2009, July 17). *Nearly half of Americans exercise less than three days a week*. Gallup. https://news.gallup.com/poll/118570/nearly-half-exercise-less-three-days-week.aspx

2. Centers for Disease Control and Prevention (CDC). (2018). National Health Statistics Reports: No. 112. U.S. Department of Health & Human Services. https://www.cdc.gov/nchs/data/nhsr/nhsr112.pdf

3. Ducharme, J. (2018, June 28). *Few Americans meet exercise guidelines: Here's what works*. TIME. https://time.com/5324940/americans-exercise-physical-activity-guidelines/

4. QuickStats: Percentage of Adults Aged ≥18 Years Who Met the Federal Guidelines for Muscle-Strengthening Physical Activity,† by Age Group and Sex — National Health Interview Survey, United States, 2020§. MMWR Morb Mortal Wkly Rep 2022;71:642. DOI: http://dx.doi.org/10.15585/mmwr.mm7118a6

5. Global Wellness Institute. (2019, October 15). *U.S. leads overall spend in $828 billion physical activity market*. https://globalwellnessinstitute.org/press-room/press-releases/us-leads-overall-spend-in-828-billion-physical-activity-market/

6. Organisation for Economic Co-operation and Development (OECD). (2019). *Health at a glance: OECD indicators*. OECD Publishing. https://www.oecd-ilibrary.org/sites/1d229f1f-en/index.html?itemId=/content/component/1d229f1f-en

7. World Health Organization (WHO). (2022). *Physical activity factsheets for the European Union member states in the WHO European region*. WHO Regional Office for Europe. https://iris.who.int/bitstream/handle/10665/353747/9789289057738-eng.pdf

8. Janssen F, Bardoutsos A, Vidra N. *Obesity Prevalence in the Long-Term Future in 18 European Countries and in the USA*. Obes Facts. 2020;13(5):514-527. doi: 10.1159/000511023. Epub 2020 Oct 19. PMID: 33075798; PMCID: PMC7670332. https://www.ncbi.nlm.nih.gov/pmc/articles/PMC7670332/

9. Eurostat. (2023). Overweight and obesity - BMI statistics. European Commission. https://ec.europa.eu/eurostat/statistics-explained/index.php?title=Overweight_and_obesity_-_BMI_statistics

10. Firth, J. (2019, November 6). *Your brain on sugar: What the science actually says*.

The Conversation. https://theconversation.com/your-brain-on-sugar-what-the-science-actually-says-126581

11. Healthy Food Guide. (2023). *The science behind our desire for salt.* https://www.healthyfood.com/advice/the-science-behind-our-desire-for-salt/

12. Goodreads. (n.d.). *A goal without a plan is just a wish.* Goodreads. https://www.goodreads.com/quotes/87476-a-goal-without-a-plan-is-just-a-wish

13. Abdelaal M, le Roux CW, Docherty NG. Morbidity and mortality associated with obesity. Ann Transl Med. 2017 Apr;5(7):161. doi: 10.21037/atm.2017.03.107. PMID: 28480197; PMCID: PMC5401682. https://www.ncbi.nlm.nih.gov/pmc/articles/PMC5401682

14. Pi-Sunyer X. *The medical risks of obesity.* Postgrad Med. 2009 Nov;121(6):21-33. doi: 10.3810/pgm.2009.11.2074. PMID: 19940414; PMCID: PMC2879283. - https://www.ncbi.nlm.nih.gov/pmc/articles/PMC2879283/

Chapter 2

1. Rodriguez Fernandez, C. (2024, December 6). *Evolutionary biology explains why we make bad long-term decisions.* Advanced Science News. https://www.advancedsciencenews.com/evolutionary-biology-explains-why-we-make-bad-long-term-decisions/

2. Zhang, Z., & Chen, W. (2019). *A systematic review of the relationship between physical activity and happiness.* Journal of Happiness Studies, 20(4), 1305–1322. https://doi.org/10.1007/s10902-018-9976-0

3. Thau, L., Gandhi, J., & Sharma, S. (2023). Physiology, *cortisol.* In StatPearls. StatPearls Publishing. Retrieved from https://www.ncbi.nlm.nih.gov/books/NBK538239/

4. Haddad, L. M., & Toney-Butler, T. J. (2023). *Empowerment.* In StatPearls. StatPearls Publishing. Retrieved from https://www.ncbi.nlm.nih.gov/books/NBK430929/

5. Bloomberg News. (2019, January 16). *The rise and fall of New Year's fitness resolutions, in 5 charts.* Bloomberg. Retrieved from https://www.bloomberg.com/news/articles/2019-01-16/here-s-how-quickly-people-ditch-weight-loss-resolutions

6. Annabel Rackham. (2023, July 15). *Why do people always wait until January to get fit?.* BBC News. Retrieved from https://www.bbc.com/news/health-67559290

7. Marion, S. (2023, January 26). *Moving past the pandemic: How fitness habits*

have changed. Health & Fitness Association. Retrieved from https://www.healthandfitness.org/improve-your-club/moving-past-the-pandemic-how-fitness-habits-have-changed/

Chapter 3

1. López-Otín C, Blasco MA, Partridge L, Serrano M, Kroemer G. *The hallmarks of aging.* Cell. 2013 Jun 6;153(6):1194-217. doi: 10.1016/j.cell.2013.05.039. PMID: 23746838; PMCID: PMC3836174. https://www.ncbi.nlm.nih.gov/pmc/articles/PMC3836174

2. Carlos López-Otín, Maria A. Blasco, Linda Partridge, Manuel Serrano, Guido Kroemer, *Hallmarks of aging: An expanding universe*, Cell, Volume 186, Issue 2, 2023, Pages 243-278, ISSN 0092-8674, https://doi.org/10.1016/j.cell.2022.11.001. https://www.sciencedirect.com/science/article/pii/S0092867422013770

3. Live Science Staff. (2009, June 22). *Brain sees tools as extensions of body.* Live Science. https://www.livescience.com/9664-brain-sees-tools-extensions-body.html

4. Power, J. D., & Schlaggar, B. L. (2017). *Neural plasticity across the lifespan.* Wiley Interdisciplinary Reviews: Developmental Biology, 6(1), e216. https://doi.org/10.1002/wdev.216

5. Maravita, A., & Iriki, A. (2004). *Tools for the body (schema).* Trends in Cognitive Sciences, 8(2), 79–86. https://doi.org/10.1016/j.tics.2003.12.008

6. Cardinali, L., Brozzoli, C., & Farnè, A. (2009). *Peripersonal space and body schema: Two labels for the same concept?* Brain Topography, 21(3–4), 252–260. https://doi.org/10.1007/s10548-009-0092-7

7. Holmes, N. P., & Spence, C. (2004). *The body schema and multisensory representation(s) of peripersonal space.* Cognitive Processing, 5(2), 94–105. https://doi.org/10.1007/s10339-004-0013-3

8. Maravita, A., Spence, C., & Driver, J. (2003). *Multisensory integration and the body schema: Close to hand and within reach.* Trends in Cognitive Sciences, 7(12), 517–523. https://doi.org/10.1016/j.tics.2003.10.015

9. Schmid, M. (2010, February 1). *To the brain, a tool is just a tool, not a hand extension.* Scientific American. https://www.scientificamerican.com/article/to-the-brain-a-tool-is-just-a-tool-not-a-hand-extension/

10. Bassolino, M., Serino, A., Ubaldi, S., & Làdavas, E. (2010). *Everyday use of the computer mouse extends peripersonal space representation.* Neuropsychologia, 48(3), 803–811. https://doi.org/10.1016/j.neuropsychologia.2009.11.009

Chapter 4

1. Michl P, Meindl T, Meister F, Born C, Engel RR, Reiser M, Hennig-Fast K. *Neurobiological underpinnings of shame and guilt: a pilot fMRI study.* Soc Cogn Affect Neurosci. 2014 Feb;9(2):150-7. doi: 10.1093/scan/nss114. Epub 2012 Oct 9. PMID: 23051901; PMCID: PMC3907920.
2. Morey RA, McCarthy G, Selgrade ES, Seth S, Nasser JD, LaBar KS. *Neural systems for guilt from actions affecting self versus others.* Neuroimage. 2012 Mar;60(1):683-92. doi: 10.1016/j.neuroimage.2011.12.069. Epub 2012 Jan 2. PMID: 22230947; PMCID: PMC3288150. https://www.ncbi.nlm.nih.gov/pmc/articles/PMC3288150/
3. Crum AJ, Langer EJ. *Mind-set matters: exercise and the placebo effect.* Psychol Sci. 2007 Feb;18(2):165-71. doi: 10.1111/j.1467-9280.2007.01867.x. PMID: 17425538. https://pubmed.ncbi.nlm.nih.gov/17425538/
4. Smith EN, Young MD, Crum AJ. *Stress, Mindsets, and Success in Navy SEALs Special Warfare Training.* Front Psychol. 2020 Jan 15;10:2962. doi: 10.3389/fpsyg.2019.02962. PMID: 32010023; PMCID: PMC6974804. https://www.ncbi.nlm.nih.gov/pmc/articles/PMC6974804/
5. Mills, Monica & Lewis, Joanna & McConnell, Daniel & Neider, Mark. (2014). *The Effects of Stress on Distance Perception.* Journal of Vision. 14. 1358. 10.1167/14.10.1358. https://www.researchgate.net/publication/265013312_The_Effects_of_Stress_on_Distance_Perception
6. Cintia Folgueira et al., *Remodeling p38 signaling in muscle controls locomotor activity via IL-15.*Sci. Adv.10,eadn5993(2024).DOI:10.1126/sciadv.adn5993
7. Wang H, Ye J. *Regulation of energy balance by inflammation: common theme in physiology and pathology.* Rev Endocr Metab Disord. 2015 Mar;16(1):47-54. doi: 10.1007/s11154-014-9306-8. PMID: 25526866; PMCID: PMC4346537. https://www.ncbi.nlm.nih.gov/pmc/articles/PMC4346537/
8. Lacourt TE, Vichaya EG, Chiu GS, Dantzer R and Heijnen CJ (2018) *The High Costs of Low-Grade Inflammation: Persistent Fatigue as a Consequence of Reduced Cellular-Energy Availability and Non-adaptive Energy Expenditure.* Front. Behav. Neurosci. 12:78. doi: 10.3389/fnbeh.2018.00078 https://www.frontiersin.org/journals/behavioral-neuroscience/articles/10.3389/fnbeh.2018.00078/full
9. Scheiber A, Mank V. *Anti-Inflammatory Diets.* [Updated 2023 Oct 28]. In: StatPearls [Internet]. Treasure Island (FL): StatPearls Publishing; 2024 Jan-. Available from: https://www.ncbi.nlm.nih.gov/books/NBK597377/

10. P. Kent Langston et al., *Regulatory T cells shield muscle mitochondria from interferon-γ–mediated damage to promote the beneficial effects of exercise.* Sci. Immunol.8,eadi5377(2023).DOI:10.1126/sciimmunol.adi5377

11. Noetel M, Sanders T, Gallardo-Gómez D, Taylor P, Del Pozo Cruz B, van den Hoek D, Smith JJ, Mahoney J, Spathis J, Moresi M, Pagano R, Pagano L, Vasconcellos R, Arnott H, Varley B, Parker P, Biddle S, Lonsdale C. *Effect of exercise for depression: systematic review and network meta-analysis of randomised controlled trials.* BMJ. 2024 Feb 14;384:e075847. doi: 10.1136/bmj-2023-075847. Erratum in: BMJ. 2024 May 28;385:q1024. doi: 10.1136/bmj. q1024. PMID: 38355154; PMCID: PMC10870815. https://pubmed. ncbi.nlm.nih.gov/38355154/

12. Sapin, D. (1979). *Stress is the number 1 killer.* Security Management, 23(5), 26–28, 30–31. Retrieved from https://www.ojp.gov/ncjrs/virtual-library/ abstracts/stress-number-1-killer

13. Childs E, de Wit H. *Regular exercise is associated with emotional resilience to acute stress in healthy adults.* Front Physiol. 2014 May 1;5:161. doi: 10.3389/ fphys.2014.00161. PMID: 24822048; PMCID: PMC4013452. https:// www.ncbi.nlm.nih.gov/pmc/articles/PMC4013452/

14. Schultchen D, Reichenberger J, Mittl T, Weh TRM, Smyth JM, Blechert J, Pollatos O. *Bidirectional relationship of stress and affect with physical activity and healthy eating.* Br J Health Psychol. 2019 May;24(2):315-333. doi: 10.1111/ bjhp.12355. Epub 2019 Jan 22. PMID: 30672069; PMCID: PMC6767465. https://www.ncbi.nlm.nih.gov/pmc/articles/PMC6767465/

15. Breit S, Kupferberg A, Rogler G, Hasler G. *Vagus Nerve as Modulator of the Brain-Gut Axis in Psychiatric and Inflammatory Disorders.* Front Psychiatry. 2018 Mar 13;9:44. doi: 10.3389/fpsyt.2018.00044. PMID: 29593576; PMCID: PMC5859128. https://www.ncbi.nlm.nih.gov/pmc/articles/ PMC5859128/

16. Ramirez JM. *The integrative role of the sigh in psychology, physiology, pathology, and neurobiology.* Prog Brain Res. 2014;209:91-129. doi: 10.1016/B978-0-444-63274-6.00006-0. PMID: 24746045; PMCID: PMC4427060. https:// www.ncbi.nlm.nih.gov/pmc/articles/PMC4427060

17. Tabung FK, Smith-Warner SA, Chavarro JE, Wu K, Fuchs CS, Hu FB, Chan AT, Willett WC, Giovannucci EL. *Development and Validation of an Empirical Dietary Inflammatory Index.* J Nutr. 2016 Aug;146(8):1560-70. doi: 10.3945/jn.115.228718. Epub 2016 Jun 29. PMID: 27358416; PMCID: PMC4958288. https://www.ncbi.nlm.nih.gov/pmc/articles/ PMC4958288/

18. Centers for Disease Control and Prevention. (n.d.). *Childhood obesity facts.*

U.S. Department of Health & Human Services. Retrieved February 5, 2025, from https://www.cdc.gov/obesity/childhood-obesity-facts/childhood-obesity-facts.html

19. Restrepo, B. J. (2022, July 5). *Adult obesity prevalence increased during the first year of the COVID-19 pandemic*. U.S. Department of Agriculture, Economic Research Service. Retrieved from https://www.ers.usda.gov/amber-waves/2022/july/adult-obesity-prevalence-increased-during-the-first-year-of-the-covid-19-pandemic/

20. World Obesity Federation. (2022). World obesity atlas 2022. Retrieved from https://www.worldobesity.org/resources/resource-library/world-obesity-atlas-2022

21. World Health Organization. (2024, March 1). *One in eight people are now living with obesity*. Retrieved from https://www.who.int/news/item/01-03-2024-one-in-eight-people-are-now-living-with-obesity

Chapter 5

1. Live Science Staff. (2009, June 22). *Brain sees tools as extensions of body*. Live Science. Retrieved from https://www.livescience.com/9664-brain-sees-tools-extensions-body.html

2. Power, J. D., & Schlaggar, B. L. (2017). *Neural plasticity across the lifespan*. Wiley Interdisciplinary Reviews: Developmental Biology, 6(1), e216. https://doi.org/10.1002/wdev.216

3. Maravita, A., & Iriki, A. (2004). *Tools for the body (schema)*. Trends in Cognitive Sciences, 8(2), 79–86. https://doi.org/10.1016/j.tics.2003.12.008

4. Cardinali, L., Brozzoli, C., & Farnè, A. (2009). *Peripersonal space and body schema: Two labels for the same concept?* Brain Topography, 21(3–4), 252–260. https://doi.org/10.1007/s10548-009-0092-7

5. Holmes, N. P., & Spence, C. (2004). *The body schema and multisensory representation(s) of peripersonal space*. Cognitive Processing, 5(2), 94–105. https://doi.org/10.1007/s10339-004-0013-3

6. Maravita, A., Spence, C., & Driver, J. (2003). *Multisensory integration and the body schema: Close to hand and within reach*. Trends in Cognitive Sciences, 7(12), 517–523. https://doi.org/10.1016/j.tics.2003.10.015

7. Schmid, M. (2010, February 1). *To the brain, a tool is just a tool, not a hand extension*. Scientific American. Retrieved from https://www.scientificamerican.com/article/to-the-brain-a-tool-is-just-a-tool-not-a-hand-extension/

8. Bassolino, M., Serino, A., Ubaldi, S., & Làdavas, E. (2010). *Everyday use of*

the computer mouse extends peripersonal space representation. Neuropsychologia, 48(3), 803–811. https://doi.org/10.1016/j.neuropsychologia.2009.11.009

9. Ejtahed HS, Mardi P, Hejrani B, Mahdavi FS, Ghoreshi B, Gohari K, Heidari-Beni M, Qorbani M. *Association between junk food consumption and mental health problems in adults: a systematic review and meta-analysis.* BMC Psychiatry. 2024 Jun 12;24(1):438. doi: 10.1186/s12888-024-05889-8. PMID: 38867156; PMCID: PMC11167869. https://www.ncbi.nlm.nih. gov/pmc/articles/PMC11167869

10. Mergenthaler P, Lindauer U, Dienel GA, Meisel A. *Sugar for the brain: the role of glucose in physiological and pathological brain function.* Trends Neurosci. 2013 Oct;36(10):587-97. doi: 10.1016/j.tins.2013.07.001. Epub 2013 Aug 20. PMID: 23968694; PMCID: PMC3900881. https://www.ncbi.nlm. nih.gov/pmc/articles/PMC3900881

11. Purves D, Augustine GJ, Fitzpatrick D, et al., editors. *Neuroscience.* 2nd edition. Sunderland (MA): Sinauer Associates; 2001. The Enteric Nervous System. Available from: https://www.ncbi.nlm.nih.gov/books/NBK11097/

12. Tai XY, Chen C, Manohar S, Husain M. *Impact of sleep duration on executive function and brain structure.* Commun Biol. 2022 Mar 3;5(1):201. doi: 10.1038/s42003-022-03123-3. PMID: 35241774; PMCID: PMC8894343. https://www.ncbi.nlm.nih.gov/pmc/articles/PMC8894343/

13. Zimmerman ME, Benasi G, Hale C, Yeung LK, Cochran J, Brickman AM, St-Onge MP. *The effects of insufficient sleep and adequate sleep on cognitive function in healthy adults.* Sleep Health. 2024 Apr;10(2):229-236. doi: 10.1016/j.sleh.2023.11.011. Epub 2024 Jan 16. PMID: 38233280; PMCID: PMC11045317. https://pubmed.ncbi.nlm.nih.gov/38233280/

14. Adolphs R. *The social brain: neural basis of social knowledge.* Annu Rev Psychol. 2009;60:693-716. doi: 10.1146/annurev.psych.60.110707.163514. PMID: 18771388; PMCID: PMC2588649. https://www.ncbi.nlm.nih.gov/pmc/articles/PMC2588649/

15. Ward, J. (2018, March 28). *We've located the part of the brain which understands social interactions.* The Conversation. https://theconversation.com/weve-located-the-part-of-the-brain-which-understands-social-interactions-93230

16. Yale School of Medicine. (2023, October 10). *Revealing communications between brain and body.* https://medicine.yale.edu/news-article/revealing-communications-between-brain-and-body/

17. Powder, J. (2021, Fall). *The gut microbiome and the brain.* Hopkins Bloomberg Public Health Magazine. https://magazine.publichealth.jhu.edu/2021/

gut-microbiome-and-brain

18. Park Kelly Jimin , Gao Yao, (2024). *Gut-brain axis and neurodegeneration: Mechanisms and therapeutic potentials.* Frontiers in Neuroscience, 18, 1481390. https://doi.org/10.3389/fnins.2024.1481390

19. AARP. (2022, March 3). *5 brain exercises that can keep your mind sharp.* https://www.aarp.org/health/brain-health/info-2022/workouts-for-brain-health.html

20. Flinders University. (2024, February 26). *Research identifies nerve endings that shed light on gut-brain communication.* Medical Xpress. https://medicalxpress.com/news/2024-02-nerve-gut-brain-communication.html

21. Anderson, S. C. (2024, January 2). *Why your brain hates junk food.* Psychology Today. https://www.psychologytoday.com/us/articles/202401/why-your-brain-hates-junk-food

Chapter 6

1. Šimić G, Tkalčić M, Vukić V, Mulc D, Španić E, Šagud M, Olucha-Bordonau FE, Vukšić M, R Hof P. *Understanding Emotions: Origins and Roles of the Amygdala.* Biomolecules. 2021 May 31;11(6):823. doi: 10.3390/biom11060823. PMID: 34072960; PMCID: PMC8228195. https://www.ncbi.nlm.nih.gov/pmc/articles/PMC8228195/

2. Dixon T. *"Emotion": The History of a Keyword in Crisis.* Emot Rev. 2012 Oct;4(4):338-344. doi: 10.1177/1754073912445814. PMID: 23459790; PMCID: PMC3573683. https://www.ncbi.nlm.nih.gov/pmc/articles/PMC3573683/

3. White MP, Elliott LR, Gascon M, Roberts B, Fleming LE. *Blue space, health and well-being: A narrative overview and synthesis of potential benefits.* Environ Res. 2020 Dec;191:110169. doi: 10.1016/j.envres.2020.110169. Epub 2020 Sep 22. PMID: 32971082. https://www.sciencedirect.com/science/article/pii/S0013935120310665?via%3Dihub

4. Williams LE, Bargh JA. *Experiencing physical warmth promotes interpersonal warmth.* Science. 2008 Oct 24;322(5901):606-7. doi: 10.1126/science.1162548. PMID: 18948544; PMCID: PMC2737341. https://www.science.org/doi/10.1126/science.1162548

5. Spada, M. (2024, July 23). *Olympians are super fit. That doesn't mean we're healthy.* The Guardian. Retrieved from https://www.theguardian.com/wellness/article/2024/jul/23/olympics-athletes-health-fitness

6. Microsoft. (n.d.). Audio Lab | *Microsoft: Inside B87.* Microsoft News.

Retrieved February 5, 2025, from https://news.microsoft.com/stories/building87/audio-lab.php

Chapter 7

1. Centre for Longitudinal Studies. (n.d.). 1970 *British Cohort Study* (BCS70). UCL Institute of Education. Retrieved February 5, 2025, from https://cls.ucl.ac.uk/cls-studies/1970-british-cohort-study/
2. Springer. (2016, October 11). *It's a myth that baby boomers have a stronger work ethic than later generations.* ScienceDaily. Retrieved from https://www.sciencedaily.com/releases/2016/10/161011135603.htm
3. Koo, J.-E., & Lee, G.-U. (2013). *The relationship of baby boomers' participation motivation in leisure sports with recovery resilience and life satisfaction.* Journal of Exercise Rehabilitation, 9(2), 263–270. https://doi.org/10.12965/jer.130009
4. Y. Dor-Ziderman, A. Lutz, A. Goldstein, *Prediction-based neural mechanisms for shielding the self from existential threat*, NeuroImage, Volume 202, 2019, 116080, ISSN 1053-8119, https://doi.org/10.1016/j.neuroimage.2019.116080.
5. Guidolin K, Jung F, Hunter S, Yan H, Englesakis M, Verderber S, Chadi S, Quereshy F. *The Influence of Exposure to Nature on Inpatient Hospital Stays: A Scoping Review.* HERD. 2024 Apr;17(2):360-375. doi: 10.1177/19375867231221559. Epub 2024 Jan 30. PMID: 38288612; PMCID: PMC11080386. https://journals.sagepub.com/doi/10.1177/19375867231221559
6. van Iperen ID, Maas J, Spronk PE. *Greenery and outdoor facilities to improve the wellbeing of critically ill patients, their families and caregivers: things to consider.* Intensive Care Med. 2023 Oct;49(10):1229-1231. doi: 10.1007/s00134-023-07185-7. Epub 2023 Aug 23. PMID: 37610484; PMCID: PMC10556109. https://pmc.ncbi.nlm.nih.gov/articles/PMC10556109/
7. George MacKerron, Susana Mourato, *Happiness is greater in natural environments*, Global Environmental Change, Volume 23, Issue 5, 2013, Pages 992-1000, ISSN 0959-3780, https://doi.org/10.1016/j.gloenvcha.2013.03.010.
8. Edmond, C., & North, M. (2023, September 28). *More than 1 in 10 people in Japan are aged 80 or over. Here's how its ageing population is reshaping the country.* World Economic Forum. Retrieved from https://www.weforum.org/stories/2023/09/elderly-oldest-population-world-japan
9. Mema E, Spain ES, Martin CK, Hill JO, Sayer RD, McInvale HD, Evans LA, Gist NH, Borowsky AD, Thomas DM. *Social influences on physical*

activity for establishing criteria leading to exercise persistence. PLoS One. 2022 Oct 19;17(10):e0274259. doi: 10.1371/journal.pone.0274259. PMID: 36260559; PMCID: PMC9581432. https://www.ncbi.nlm.nih.gov/pmc/articles/PMC9581432/

10. Söderström, T. (2021). *A 20-year analysis of motives and training patterns of Swedish gym-goers.* Annals of Leisure Research, 26(4), 521–544. https://doi.org/10.1080/11745398.2021.2010223

Index